Making Sense of the Pediatric EEG

Most neurologists, fellows, and residents are familiar with adult electroencephalogram (EEG) but have not developed a similar understanding of pediatric EEG. There are fewer resources covering pediatric electroencephalography, and existing books are either too comprehensive or lack the main details that differentiate the EEG in childhood. This accessible text includes the most recent classification and nomenclature published by the International League Against Epilepsy. It provides a practical and well-illustrated text of value to residents, fellows, and neurologists in need of an update on pediatric EEG.

Making Sense of the Pediatric EEG

Edited by

Maria Augusta Montenegro, MD, PhD

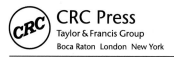

CRC Press
Taylor & Francis Group
Boca Raton London New York

CRC Press is an imprint of the
Taylor & Francis Group, an **informa** business

First edition published 2024
by CRC Press
6000 Broken Sound Parkway NW, Suite 300, Boca Raton, FL 33487–2742

and by CRC Press
4 Park Square, Milton Park, Abingdon, Oxon, OX14 4RN

CRC Press is an imprint of Taylor & Francis Group, LLC

© 2024 selection and editorial matter, Maria Augusta Montenegro;
individual chapters, the contributors

ISBN: 9781032486093 (hbk)
ISBN: 9781032486079 (pbk)
ISBN: 9781003389866 (ebk)

DOI: 10.1201/b23339

Typeset in Minion
by KnowledgeWorks Global Ltd.

Contents

Preface

Making Sense of the Pediatric EEG was written for medical students, residents, and fellows. It was also written for neurologists who treat children with epilepsy but are not epileptologists.

The book is richly illustrated, and the text provides a systematic approach to pediatric electroencephalography, including the maturational changes seen throughout childhood, and the recent updates in the terminology of EEG and pediatric epilepsy. There are chapters dedicated to neonatal seizures, epileptic encephalopathies, and the focal and generalized epilepsy syndromes most frequently seen in childhood.

We hope that the simple and clear approach provided by the book will help the reader not only make sense of pediatric electroencephalography but also enjoy reading it.

Maria Augusta Montenegro, MD, PhD
Rady Children's Hospital
University of California San Diego

About the author

Maria Augusta Montenegro, MD, PhD, is a pediatric neurologist/epileptologist originally from Brazil. Following her residency program and PhD, she undertook a post-doctorate fellowship in New York (Columbia University) and Boston (Herscot Center for Tuberous Sclerosis Complex/MGH).

Maria was the chief of pediatric neurology at the University of Campinas (Brazil), and in 2022, she moved to the United States to work at Rady Children's Hospital/UCSD as a pediatric neurologist/epileptologist. Maria has written several books and scientific chapters.

Contributors

All the esteemed contributors to this book are part of the faculty at Rady's Children's Hospital, San Diego, CA, USA, and its affiliate University of California San Diego School of Medicine.

Michaela A. Castello, MD, PhD

Aliya Frederick, MD, PhD

Jeffrey Gold, MD, PhD

Olivia Kim-McManus, MD

Mark Nespeca, MD

Jong M. Rho, MD

Neggy Rismanchi, MD, PhD

Shifteh Sattar, MD

Brittany Sprigg, MD

Abbreviations and acronyms

BETS	benign epileptiform transient of sleep
BIPDs	bilateral independent periodic discharges
BIRD	brief interictal/ictal rhythmic discharges
BRD	brief rhythmic discharge
COVE	childhood occipital visual epilepsy
DEE	developmental and epileptic encephalopathies
DEE/SWAS	developmental and epileptic encephalopathy with spike-wave activation in sleep
EEG	electroencephalogram
EIDEE	early -infantile developmental and epileptic encephalopathy
EKG	electrocardiogram
EPSP	excitatory postsynaptic potential
GPD	generalized periodic discharge
GTC	generalized tonic clonic
IPSP	inhibitory postsynaptic potentials
JME	juvenile myoclonic epilepsy
LPD	lateralized periodic discharge
MfPD	multifocal periodic discharge
POLE	photosensitive occipital lobe epilepsy
POSTS	positive occipital sharp transient of sleep
REM	rapid eye movement
SeLAS	self-limited epilepsy with autonomic seizures
SeLECTS	self-limited epilepsy with centrotemporal spikes
SeLFNIE	self-limited familial neonatal-infantile epilepsy
SeLIE	self-limited (familial) infantile epilepsy
SeLNE	self-limited neonatal epilepsy
SREDA	subclinical rhythmic electrographic discharge of adults

CHAPTER 1

Basic principles

Michaela A. Castello, MD, PhD

Maria Augusta Montenegro, MD, PhD

Jong M. Rho, MD

Electrical impulses flow between neurons via action potentials that initiate neurotransmission at both excitatory and inhibitory synapses in the central nervous system (CNS), and ion channels largely mediate the electrophysiological changes necessary to transmit signals from one neuron to another. The brain is a highly complex network of interlinked cells (both neurons and glia), and the net (summated) activity is dependent on the balance and timing of inhibitory and excitatory influences. The voltage changes at a microscopic level are reflected in either excitatory postsynaptic potentials (EPSPs) or inhibitory postsynaptic potentials (IPSPs), and the combined effects of these electrophysiological changes determines outputs such as a depolarization of the cellular membrane potential sufficient to trigger an action potential.

- EPSP: Flow of *positive* ions into the neuron or flow of *negative* ions out of the neuron.
- IPSP: Flow of *negative* ions into the neuron or flow of *positive* ions out of the neuron.

The neuronal resting membrane potential is approximately -70 mV. An action potential is generated by the initial depolarization mediated by Ca^{2+} influx into the neuron, which increases its cell membrane potential to cross the threshold

DOI: 10.1201/b23339-1

for voltage-gated sodium channel activation—resulting in the upstroke of the action potential. Subsequently, K⁺ efflux and Cl⁻ influx into the neuron cause neuronal repolarization (and transitory hyperpolarization). The action potential activates the presynaptic exocytosis mechanisms to release neurotransmitters into the synaptic cleft, which then exert their activity on postsynaptic, presynaptic and astrocytic targets. In the case of glutamate, the principal excitatory neurotransmitter in the CNS, both ionotropic (*N*-methyl-D-aspartate [NMDA] and α-amino-3-hydroxy-5-methyl-4-isoxazolepropionic acid [AMPA]) or metabotropic receptors are activated downstream. In addition to calcium influx into the postsynaptic terminal, these changes trigger further consequences of synaptic neurotransmission, including action potential propagation (**Figure 1.1**).

The electrical activity captured by the electroencephalogram (EEG) is generated by a population of cortical pyramidal neurons that form a dipole perpendicular to the cortical surface (Gloor, 1977). Specifically, the EEG records the extracellular electrical activity from a large number of cortical pyramidal neurons representing the *sum* (i.e., superposition) of both EPSPs and IPSPs. Because of this, a large number of neurons are required to generate enough electrical activity that can be recorded by the EEG electrode.

In 1965, Cooper et al proposed that a minimum of 6 cm² of cortical surface area of neurons was required (Cooper *et al.*, 1965) to generate an epileptiform discharge, which is likely an underestimate of the actual cortical surface needed to produce spikes that can be detected by the EEG. More recent studies conducted with

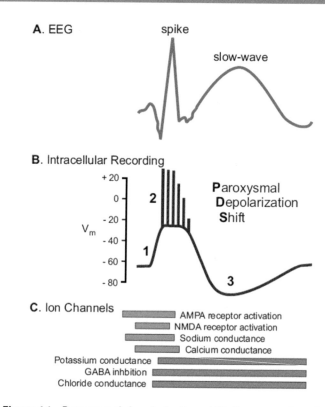

Figure 1.1   Paroxysmal depolarization shift. Representation of the (A) EEG, (B) intracellular recording, and (C) ion channels activation. Note that the spike/sharp wave does not represent the action potential itself, it is the summation of the electrical activity generated by a group of neurons during depolarization, followed by a slow wave that represents the hyperpolarization phase.

modern recording methods indicated that 6 cm^2 of synchronous cerebral depolarization rarely generated scalp-recordable EEG interictal spikes, and instead indicated that ≥10 cm^2 is likely needed (Tao *et al.*, 2005).

The recorded activity shown by scalp EEG consists of a spike (or sharp wave) that represents the electrical activity generated by a group of neurons during depolarization, followed by a slow wave that represents the hyperpolarization phase.

ELECTRODES

All electrodes must be composed of the same material, the most often being gold, silver, or chloride. The EEG setup recommended by the American Clinical Neurophysiology Society consists of 21 electrodes (19 in the scalp and one in each ear) placed according to the 10–20 configuration (**Figure 1.2**; Sinha *et al.*, 2016). The nomenclature describing each electrode is standardized: Midline electrodes are labeled "z," while the other electrodes are numbered with increasing values the further they are placed away from the midline. By convention, odd numbers are on the left and even numbers are on the right. In addition to a number, each electrode receives a letter corresponding to the approximate underlying anatomical area (broadly, the lobes of the brain), e.g., the F4 electrode is the right frontal, while O1 is left occipital (Acharya *et al.*, 2016). Before recording the EEG, each electrode should be tested for opposition to electrical flow (i.e., impedance), which cannot exceed 5,000 Ohms.

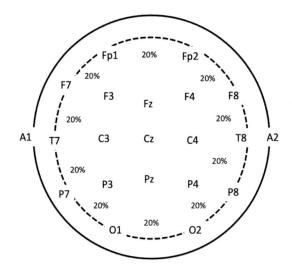

Figure 1.2   The 10–20 system of electrode placement. This system was designed to maintain a fixed relative distance of 10% or 20% of the total head measurement between each electrode. This enables a consistent relationship between electrodes and the underlying cortical areas.

CHANNELS AND MONTAGES

The EEG records the difference in voltage (i.e., the potential difference) between two electrodes (each representing a large group of neurons). Each EEG channel ("line of the EEG" on a screen or paper tracing) registers the difference between two points. The goal is to simultaneously record as many regions as possible to determine if there are any abnormal voltage oscillations or patterns that might indicate an underlying brain dysfunction or a susceptibility to seizure generation.

The minimum number of channels required by the American Clinical Neurophysiology Society is 16, but additional channels can be included to enable recordings from more cortical areas or physiologic parameters such as EKG or eye movements (Sinha *et al.,* 2016). Much like the electrodes themselves, channels are organized into montages that must adhere to a standardized pattern: Channels representing anterior electrodes are placed above the channels

representing posterior regions, and left electrodes are placed above the right electrodes (Acharya *et al.,* 2016). The relative distance between electrodes should remain the same, while the electrodes are placed to allow comparison between each homologous area.

There are two main types of montages: Bipolar and referential. Bipolar montages record the potential difference between two different sequential electrodes; that is, the electrode that enters input 2 of the first channel also enters input 1 of the next channel (**Figure 1.3**). These sequences must be arranged

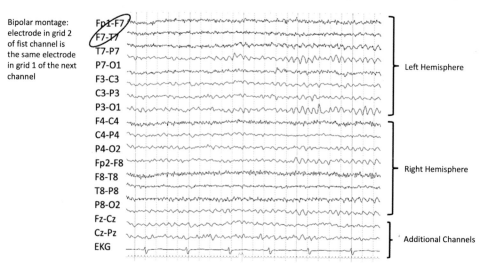

Figure 1.3　EEG montage. Note that the anterior electrodes are placed above the posterior electrodes and the left-sided (i.e., odd numbers) electrodes are placed above the right-sided (i.e., even numbers) electrodes. The areas covered in the left hemisphere are homologous to those covered by electrodes in the right hemisphere.

longitudinally or transversely. Referential montages record the potential difference between each electrode and a common value, which enables to use of the wave amplitude to establish the source of the discharge (i.e., the electrode recording the highest amplitude is closer to the source or the epileptogenic area).

Each montage records the brain activity from a different angle, as though one were to view an object from different directions. Different montages provide more complementary and confirmative information, which enables better lateralization and localization of electrographic findings (**Figures 1.4–1.6**).

Longitudinal			Transverse	
Fp1-F7	Fp1-F3	Fp1-F7	F7-Fp1	F7-Fp1
F7-T7	F3-C3	F7-T7	Fp1-Fp2	F7-F3
T7-P7	C3-P3	T7-P7	Fp2-F8	F3-Fz
P7-O1	P3-O1	P7-O1	Fz-F3	Fz-F4
Fp1-F3	Fp2-F4	Fp2-F8	F3-Fz	F4-F8
F3-C3	F4-C4	F8-T8	Fz-F4	A1-T7
C3-P3	C4-P4	T8-P8	F4-F8	T7-C3
P3-O1	P4-O2	P8-O2	T7-C3	C3-Cz
Fp2-F4	Fp1-F7	Fp1-F3	C3-Cz	Cz-C4
F4-C4	F7-T7	F3-C3	Cz-C4	C4-T8
C4-P4	T7-P7	C3-P3	C4-T8	T8-A2
P4-O2	P7-O1	P3-O1	P7-P3	P7-P3
Fp2-F8	Fp2-F8	Fp2-F4	P3-Pz	P3-Pz
F8-T8	F8-T8	F4-C4	Pz-P4	Pz-P4
T8-P8	T8-P8	C4-P4	P4-P8	P4-P8
P8-O2	P8-O2	P4-O2	O1-O2	O1-O2
ECG	ECG	ECG	ECG	ECG

Figure 1.5   EEG montage. Frequently used longitudinal and transverse montages. (From Acharya et al., 2016.)

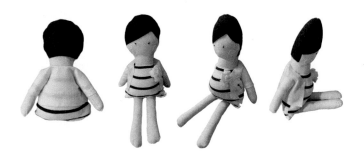

Figure 1.4   Montages. Each montage records the brain activity from a different angle as if one was to observe an object from different directions.

RECORDING THE EEG

The voltage underneath each electrode is captured and sent to the EEG machine, which:

a. Filters the activity that is not important for the EEG recording.

b. Excludes signals that appear simultaneously in all electrodes, like the EKG for example (common mode rejection).

A

B

C

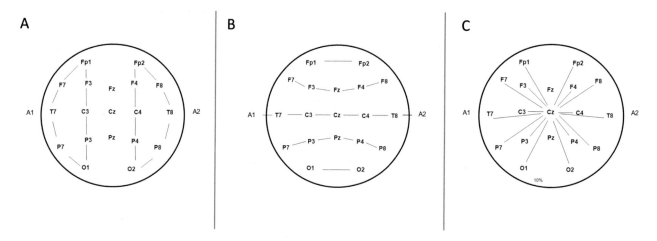

Figure 1.6 Examples of bipolar and referential montages. In bipolar montages, the electrodes are sequentially arranged (A) longitudinally or (B) transversely. (C) Referential montages usually use the average, Cz, or ear electrodes (A1 for left hemisphere electrodes and A2 for right hemisphere electrodes).

c. Calculates the potential difference between two electrodes.

d. Amplifies its voltage.

e. Displays it as a graph of voltage *versus* time (**Figure 1.7**).

In each channel, the deflection will go downward or upward depending on the potential *difference* between the two electrodes. If the voltage in the first electrode is more positive than the voltage in the second electrode, the channel will record a downward deflection, and if the voltage in the first electrode is more negative than the voltage in the second electrode, the channel will record an upward deflection (**Figure 1.8**).

FILTERS

There are three types of filters: High-frequency (blocks waves above the established frequency), low-frequency (blocks waves below the established frequency), and notch filters (blocks only a specific frequency, typically 60 Hz activity from the building's

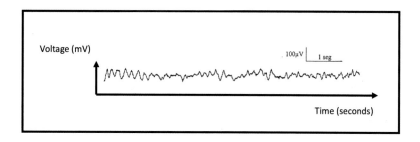

Figure 1.7 EEG recording. The EEG machine filters and amplifies the electrical activity of the brain. Each channel of the EEG represents the potential difference recorded and plotted as a graph of voltage *versus* time.

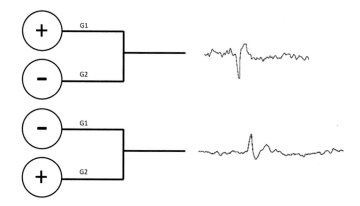

Figure 1.8 Wave polarity. The wave polarity depends on the potential difference between grid 1 and grid 2. If grid 1 is less negative than grid 2, it will cause a downward deflection. If grid 1 is more negative than grid 2, it will cause an upward deflection.

electrical current). The low-frequency filter is usually set at 1 Hz and the high-frequency filter at 70 Hz. This interval (1–70 Hz) includes the normal and abnormal frequencies generated by the brain (**Figure 1.9**):

- Posterior dominant rhythm (6–13 Hz).
- N1, N2, N3 sleep stages (2–7 Hz).
- REM sleep (8–10 Hz).
- Spikes (15–20 Hz).
- Sharp waves (5–14 Hz).
- Spike-wave complexes (2–6 Hz), theta and delta waves, etc.

Although the cutoff of the high and low-frequency filters can be changed, it should be done only by experienced

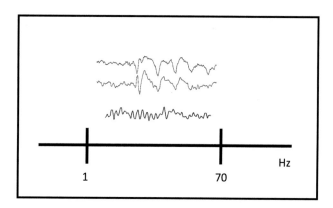

Figure 1.9   High- and low-frequency filter settings. The frequencies of the most important normal and abnormal electrical discharges generated by the brain range between 1 and 70 Hz.

neurophysiologists because important normal and abnormal waves can be distorted or attenuated. The notch filter (60 Hz in the United States) should be used when there is too much fast activity due to electrical current, especially in recordings performed in the intensive care unit setting where several electronic devices may be connected to the patient (**Figure 1.10**).

The time constant (i.e., the elapsed time required for the current to decay to 36.8% of its value, or the time that the capacitor takes to recharge 63.2% of its final value) is another important EEG

parameter that should be changed only by experienced neurophysiologists. It is usually set at 0.3, but small modifications can change the wave morphology to the point of compromising the EEG interpretation (**Figure 1.11**).

TYPE OF WAVES RECORDED

The EEG records mostly normal discharges, but occasionally abnormal waves can be identified. Each wave is classified according to its frequency (cycles per second, or Hz): Alpha, beta, theta, or delta (**Figure 1.12**). In addition, the abnormalities should also be classified according to their meaning: Epileptiform or non-epileptiform.

Epileptiform discharges are associated with increased cortical excitability and a higher risk of seizures arising from that area. Non-epileptiform abnormalities are associated with transitory or permanent dysfunction but do not necessarily signify an increased risk of seizures arising from that area. **Table 1.1** and **Figure 1.13** show the characteristics that help to differentiate an epileptiform wave from the normal background.

Epileptiform discharges are classified as spikes (<70 μV), sharp waves (70–200 μV), spike-wave complexes, or sharp-wave complexes (**Figure 1.14**). The spike-wave complexes and sharp-wave complexes can be regular or irregular, and their frequency can also be measured (**Figures 1.15–1.17**).

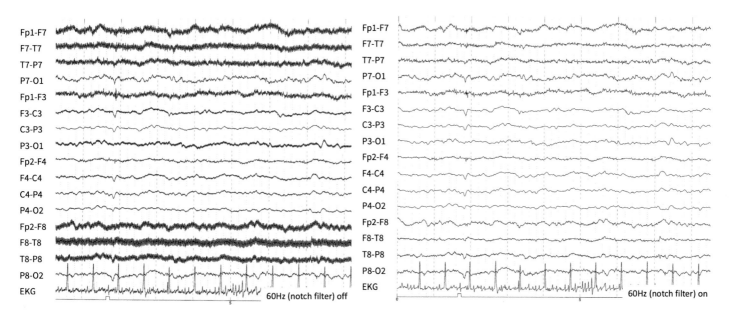

Figure 1.10   The 60 Hz (notch) filter. Difference of the EEG recording according to electric current interference. Note that when the notch (60 Hz) filter is on (right), there is a great improvement in the electric current artifact.

SENSITIVITY

The sensitivity of the EEG is the ratio of microvolts per millimeter, and it can be adjusted to either increase or reduce the height of waves during analysis. A sensitivity of 10 means that 1 mm is equal to 10 µV. The sensitivity is usually set at 7, but in children with high-amplitude epileptiform abnormalities (e.g., hypsarrhythmia), the sensitivity should be increased to 10, 15, or even 20. Increasing the sensitivity produces a decrease in wave amplitude (**Figure 1.18**).

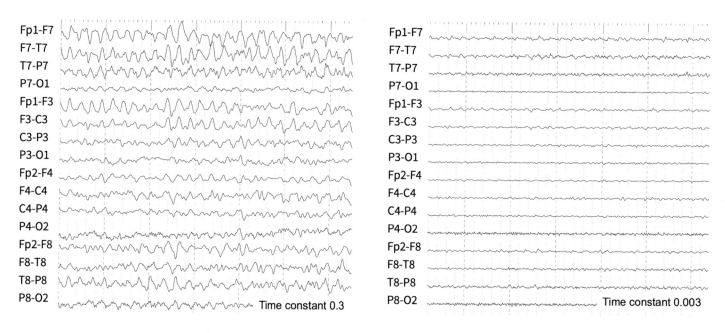

Figure 1.11   Time constant. Note the difference in the appearance of EEG signals according to the time constant setting in the same EEG sample. The recording on the left has a time constant of 0.3 (most commonly used); but if the time constant is changed to 0.003 (right), the same recording looks completely different, with severe distortion of the waves.

LOCALIZATION OF THE DISCHARGES

The brain is a volume conductor (i.e., a material capable of conducting electric current); therefore, if there is a difference in voltage between two points, it will lead to the flow of current.

The current strength varies greatly in different areas within the same volume conductor, and each EEG channel records the potential difference from a restricted area. The goal is to simultaneously record as many regions as possible; therefore, under

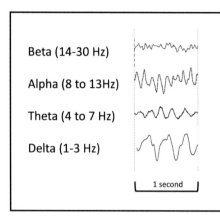

Figure 1.12   Types of EEG waves. Classification of waves according to their frequency.

Table 1.1   Characteristics that help classify a wave as epileptiform or non-epileptiform

Characteristics	Epileptiform discharge	Non-epileptiform discharge
Symmetry	Asymmetric	Symmetric
Followed by a slow wave	Frequently	No
Morphology	Biphasic or triphasic	Monophasic
Relationship with the background	Stands out	Blends in
Recorded by nearby channels (forms a field)	Yes	No

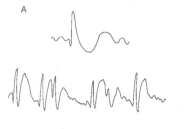

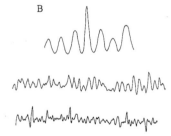

Figure 1.13   Epileptiform *versus* non-epileptiform waves. (A) Epileptiform wave: Note the asymmetrical angulation between the two upward and downward components of the spike. The spike is followed by a slow wave, has a triphasic morphology, and stands out from the background. (B) Normal background: Note the symmetric angulation of the upward and downward components of the wave. There is no subsequent slow wave, it has a monophasic appearance, and it does not stand out from the background. (Reproduced from Montenegro *et al.*, 2022; with permission.)

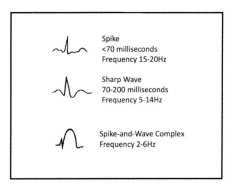

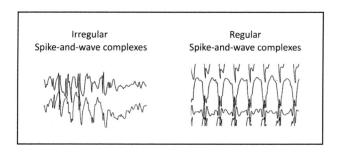

Figure 1.14 **Types of epileptiform discharges**. Note the morphology, frequency, and duration of each type of epileptiform activity: Spikes, sharp waves, and spike-wave complexes.

Figure 1.16 **Type of spike-wave complex**. Classification of spike-wave complexes according to their morphology: Irregular (different morphology) and regular (same morphology in each channel).

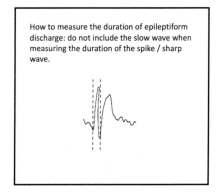

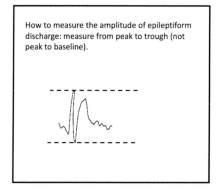

Figure 1.15 **Wave measurements**. The duration of the spike or sharp wave should be measured without including the following slow wave. The amplitude of the wave should be measured from peak to trough.

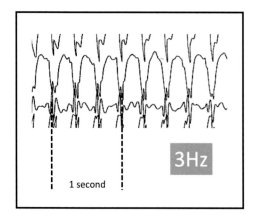

Figure 1.17 Spike and wave complex. This figure shows how to measure the frequency of spike-wave complexes.

current practice, the EEG study usually involves a minimum of 16 channels.

To localize the source of abnormal discharge, it is important to note that if two electrodes are in areas with the same voltage, they will not register any difference in potential (even if they are very close to the source). However, two electrodes with very different voltages will record a large potential, even if they are far from the source (Gloor, 1977).

This basic principle is very important in localizing an epileptiform discharge. In bipolar montages, the channel that records the potential with the highest amplitude may not represent the

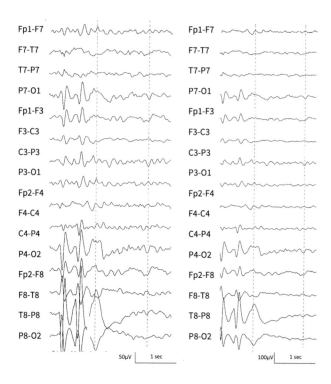

Figure 1.18 Sensitivity. Same EEG recording with different sensitivities. Increasing the sensitivity causes a decrease in amplitude.

place of maximum electrical activity; therefore, localization should be based on phase reversal or equipotentiality (no difference between two electrodes). Amplitude should be considered as one of the localization parameters only on referential montages (**Figures 1.19–1.21**).

CALIBRATION

Calibration is performed by applying the same known voltage to every channel to make sure that each channel responds equally to the applied voltage. In biological calibration, a fronto-occipital derivation should be used (Sinha *et al.*, 2016). It should be performed for at least 10 seconds at the beginning and end of every EEG recording (**Figures 1.22–1.24**).

Finally, minimum technical requirements should be followed when recording an EEG (**Table 1.2**).

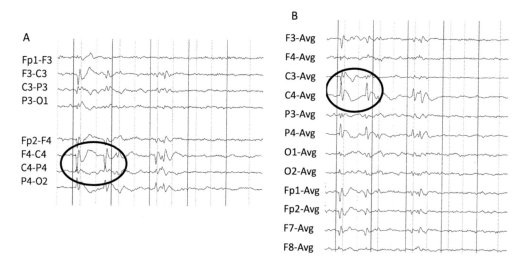

Figure 1.19   Bipolar *versus* referential montages. Same EEG recording using a bipolar and a referential montage. Note that in the bipolar montage (A), the area of maximum negativity is identified by the phase reversal (C4 electrode, almost equipotential on C4-P4); and in the referential montage (B), the same region (C4 electrode) is identified as the area of maximum negativity by the higher amplitude.

A

Fp1-F7
F7-T7
T7-P7
P7-O1

Fp1-F3
F3-C3
C3-P3
P3-O1

Fp2-F4
F4-C4
C4-P4
P4-O2

Fp2-F8
F8-T8
T8-P8
P8-O2

B

F3-Avg
F4-Avg
C3-Avg
C4-Avg
P3-Avg
P4-Avg
O1-Avg
O2-Avg
Fp1-Avg
Fp2-Avg
F7-Avg
F8-Avg
T7-Avg
T8-Avg
P7-Avg
P8-Avg

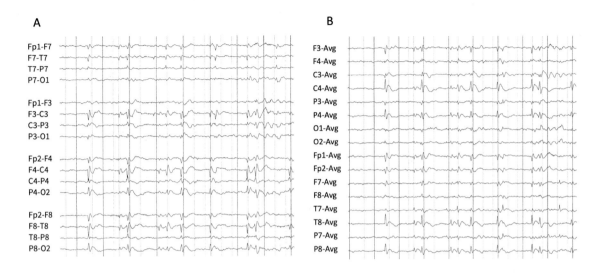

Figure 1.20 Bipolar *versus* referential montages. EEG of a boy with self-limited epilepsy with centrotemporal spikes showing very frequent sharp waves followed by slow waves in the centro-temporo-parietal head regions. Note that in the bipolar montage (A), the area of maximum negativity is identified by the phase reversal, while in the referential montage (B), the same area is identified by the higher amplitude. Also, note that in the referential montage there is a shift in the polarity in the frontal electrodes (horizontal dipole).

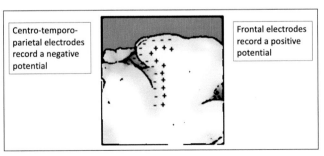

Centro-temporo-parietal electrodes record a negative potential

Frontal electrodes record a positive potential

Figure 1.21 Horizontal dipole. Referential montages enable the recording of horizontal dipoles, showing the negative (posterior electrodes) and positive (anterior electrodes, usually frontal areas) voltages of the dipole. It occurs because the focus is deep in the sulci, with neurons parallel to the scalp. It will be seen as a positive polarity wave (sharp wave "downward") at the anterior electrodes, and as a negative polarity wave (sharp wave "upward") in the more posterior electrodes.

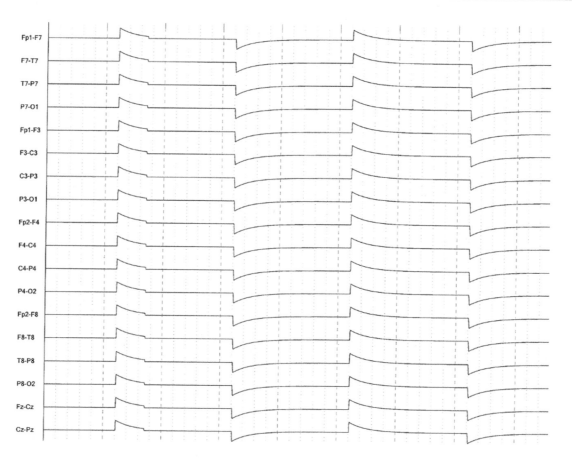

Figure 1.22 Calibration. Note that during calibration, the recording in every channel should be exactly the same.

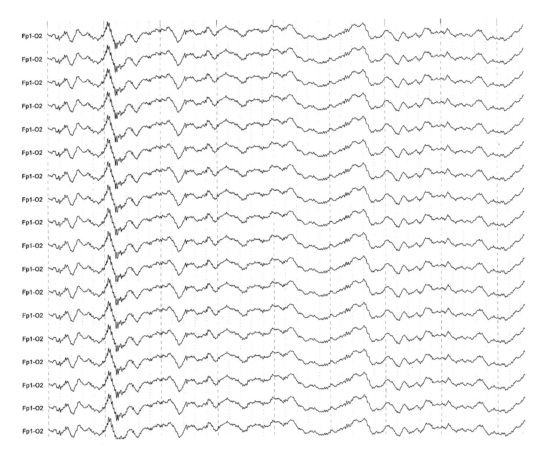

Figure 1.23 Biological calibration. In biological calibration, the most common derivation used is the fronto-occipital (Fp1-O2).

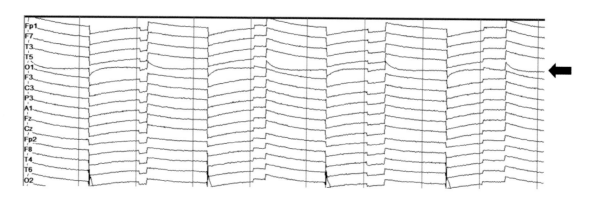

Figure 1.24   Abnormal calibration. EEG during calibration showing abnormal 6th channel (arrow). (Courtesy: Jose Amador.)

Table 1.2   Minimal technical requirements for recording the EEG

Parameter	Minimum technical requirement
Number of electrodes	At least 21
Number of channels	At least 16
Electrode placement	10–20 system
Duration of the EEG	At least 20 minutes
Type of electrodes	Silver, chloride, gold disk electrodes Needle electrodes are not recommended
Montages	At least 1 longitudinal bipolar, 1 transverse and 1 referential montage
High-frequency filter	70 Hz
Low-frequency filter	1 Hz
Time constant	0.3
60 Hz (notch) filter	Should be used only when other measures to reduce electrical current fails
Intermittent photic stimulation	30 cm from patient's face, before hyperventilation or at least 3 minutes after ending of hyperventilation Stop if a seizure is triggered
Hyperventilation	3 minutes Stop if a seizure is triggered

REFERENCES

Acharya JN, Hani AJ, Thirumala PD, Tsuchida TN. American Clinical Neurophysiology Society Guideline 3: A Proposal for Standard Montages to be used in Clinical EEG. J Clin Neurophysiol 2016;33:312–16.

Cooper R, Winter AL, Crow HJ, et al. Comparison of Subcortical, Cortical and Scalp Activity using Chronically Indwelling Electrodes in Man. Electroencephalogr Clin Neurophysiol 1965;18:217–28.

Gloor P. Application of Volume Conductor Principles to Montage Design. Am J EEG Technol 1977;17:5–20.

Montenegro MA, Cendes F, Guerreiro MM, Guerreiro CAM. EEG na Pratica Clinica. Rio de Janeiro: Thieme-Revinter; 2022.

Sinha SR, Sullivan L, Sabau D, et al. American Clinical Neurophysiology Society Guideline 1: Minimum Technical Requirements for Performing Clinical Electroencephalography. J Clin Neurophysiol 2016;33:301–07.

Tao JX, Ray A, Hawes-Ebersole S, Ebersole JS. Intracranial EEG Substrates of Scalp EEG Interictal Spikes. Epilepsia 2005;46:669–76.

CHAPTER 2

Artifacts

Maria Augusta Montenegro, MD, PhD

Artifacts are caused by interference from numerous sources such as muscle, heart, electric current, monitors, movement, etc. They are not generated by the brain and its morphology may cause misinterpretation of the EEG or obscure the recording to the point that it is impossible to read (Fisch, 1999).

EEG artifacts are classified as physiological and non-physiological, according to the type of extracerebral interference. Physiological artifacts are generated by the patient's body: Heart, muscle, eye movement, blinking, sweating, etc. Non-physiological artifacts are generated by external factors, such as electrodes, wires, electric current, etc. (Hughes, 1994; Tyner *et al.*, 1983). The most common EEG artifacts are described in **Table 2.1** (**Figures 2.1–2.25**).

The identification of artifacts by the technician is important because once the artifact source is identified, it can be corrected during the EEG recording (Ebersole & Pedley, 2003; Fisch, 1999). In addition, the technician can add valuable information by annotating information such as patient movement, crying, yawning, sucking a pacifier, patting on the child's back to keep the child calm, etc.

DOI: 10.1201/b23339-2

Table 2.1   Most common types of EEG artifacts

Type of artifact	Characteristics
Electrocardiogram artifact	Rhythmic sharp waves that coincide with the electrocardiogram (EKG).
Ballistocardiographic artifact	Medium- to high-amplitude slow wave affecting several channels. It is caused by the movement of the head, electrodes, or electrode wires as the heart beats, and it is more frequently seen in patients with electrocerebral inactivity.
Cardiac pacemaker artifact	High-amplitude spike time-locked with the pacemaker spike preceding the EKG.
Pulse artifact	Slow wave caused by electrode placement over an artery. It is recorded approximately 200 ms after the EKG, and usually affects a single electrode.
Body movement artifact	Chaotic and unpredictable changes in the recording caused by the patient's movement. As the patient moves, it shakes the electrode wires.
Muscle artifact	High-frequency spikes produced by the scalp muscles (electromyography), more frequently recorded by the frontotemporal electrodes. It can be rhythmic, especially when the patient is eating/chewing/sucking pacifier.
Blinking artifact	High-amplitude upward (eye opening) or downward (eye closure) slow wave. The cornea is positively charged, and the retina is negatively charged (which functions as a dipole). Vertical eye movements affect mostly the Fp1 and Fp2 electrodes.
Horizontal eye movement artifact	High-amplitude positive potential affecting the electrode closer to the direction of eye gaze, and negative potential in the opposite side (positive potential in F8 when looking to the right, and positive potential in F7 if looking to the left).
Lateral *rectus* spike	Spike overriding the slow wave caused by the lateral eye movement, recorded in the same side as is directed. It is best recorded by F7 or F8. It is the lateral *rectus* muscle EMG recorded during lateral gaze.
Eyelid flutter artifact	High-amplitude 3-6 Hz slow waves, better seen in Fp1 and Fp2 electrodes, usually lasting several seconds.
REM artifact	Frequent, semi-rhythmic, bilateral horizontal eye movements seen during REM sleep.
Glossokinetic artifact	High-amplitude slow wave, more evident in the frontotemporal electrodes. The tip of the tongue is negatively charged, and the base of the tongue is positively charged (which functions as a dipole). It is caused by the tongue movement while talking.
Sweating artifact	High-amplitude baseline oscillations caused by sweating, which alters the electrode impedance. It can be reduced by cooling the room.
Salt bridge artifact	Low amplitude discharges in one channel (almost no potential difference) caused by sweat "connecting" two adjacent electrodes (usually a pillowcase soaked in sweat or excessive electrode paste).
Electrode compression artifact	Slow (or sharply contoured) wave that resembles pulse artifact. It happens when something compresses the electrode (usually the patient's head). Rhythmic movements can produce waves that are difficult to distinguish from an electrographic seizure.
Electrode artifact	High-amplitude positive potential with steep component followed by a gradual return to the baseline.
Electric current artifact	60 Hz spikes caused by electrical current. It is seen when the electrode impedance is too high, or the ground electrode is not properly placed on the patient. It can be filtered by the 60 Hz (notch) filter.

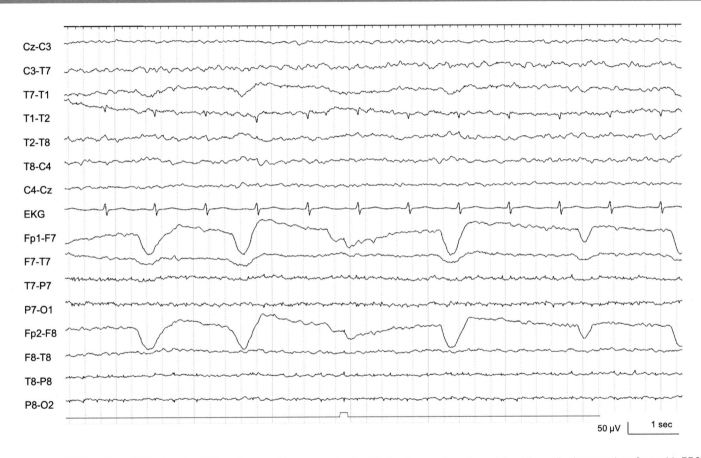

Figure 2.1   EKG artifact. EEG showing EKG artifacts, which are easily identified as being of cardiac origin and usually does not interfere with EEG reading. Also note blinking artifacts on the 9th and 13th channels.

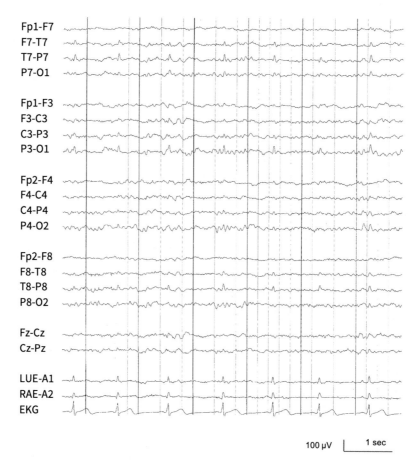

100 μV   1 sec

Figure 2.2   EKG artifact. EEG showing EKG artifacts, which are easily identified as being of cardiac origin and usually do not interfere with EEG reading.

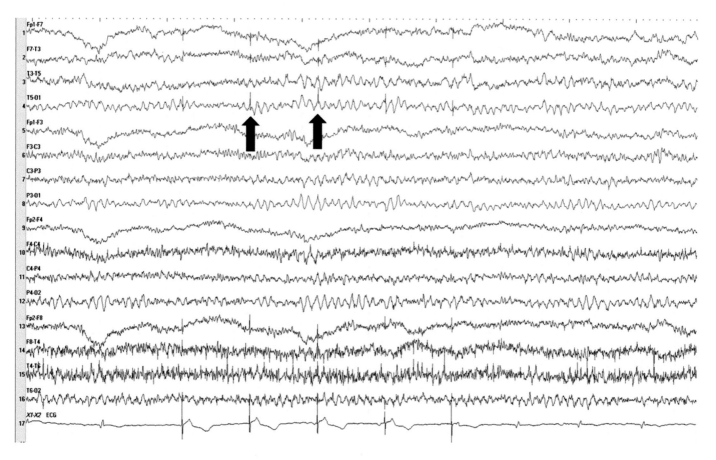

Figure 2.3 Cardiac pacemaker artifact. EEG showing high-amplitude spike (arrows) associated with cardiac pacemaker artifacts. (Reprinted from Montenegro *et al.*, 2022; with permission.)

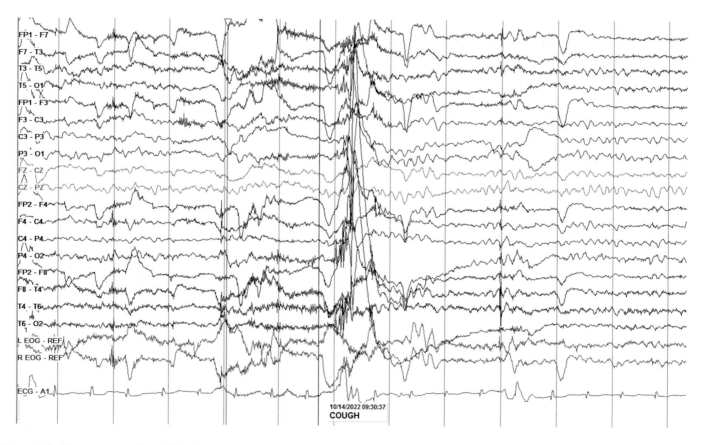

Figure 2.4 Movement artifact. EEG showing high-amplitude waves due to patient movement (cough), which causes movement of the electrode wires and interference with the recording.

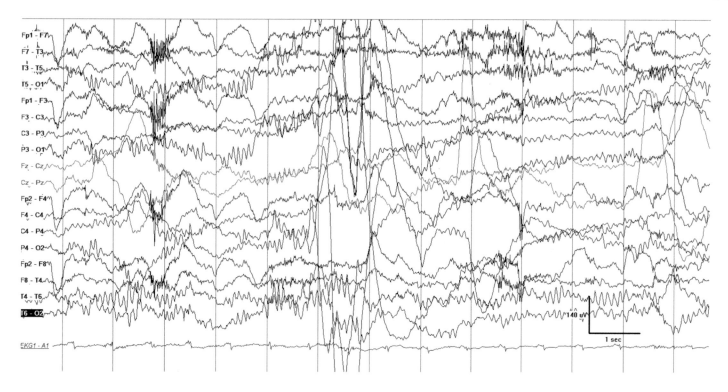

Figure 2.5 Movement artifact. EEG showing random, chaotic, unpredictable high-amplitude waves due to patient movement, which causes movement of the electrodes, electrodes wires, and interference with the recording.

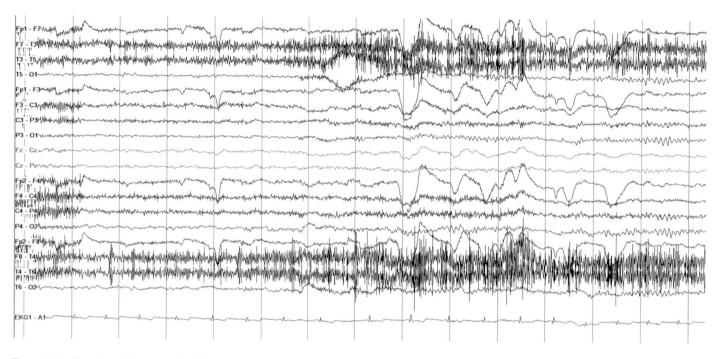

Figure 2.6　Muscle artifact. Awake EEG showing medium to high-amplitude spikes, more prominent in both temporal regions, caused by muscle contraction. (Courtesy: Joseph Zuniga.)

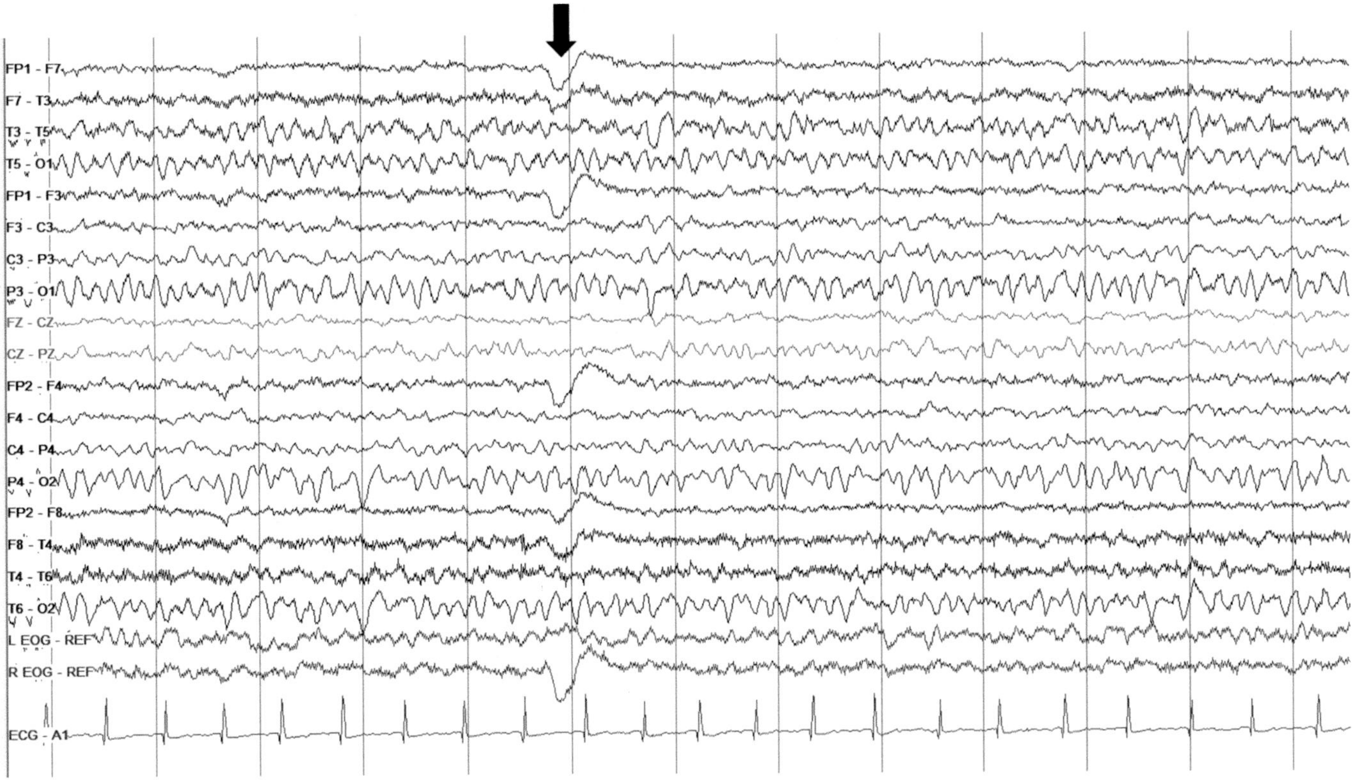

Figure 2.7 Blinking artifact. EEG showing high-amplitude sharply contoured wave in the frontal regions caused by blinking (arrow). It is caused because the cornea is positively charged and the retina is negatively charged (which functions as a dipole), and the vertical movement of the eye is recorded mostly by the Fp1 and Fp2 electrodes. During eye-opening, the cornea moves away from Fp1/Fp2 electrode, making it more negative than F3/F4 or F7/F8, causing an upward deflection. During eye closure, the cornea moves toward Fp1/Fp2, making it more positive than F3/F4 or F7/F8, producing a downward deflection. (Courtesy: Maria Warren.)

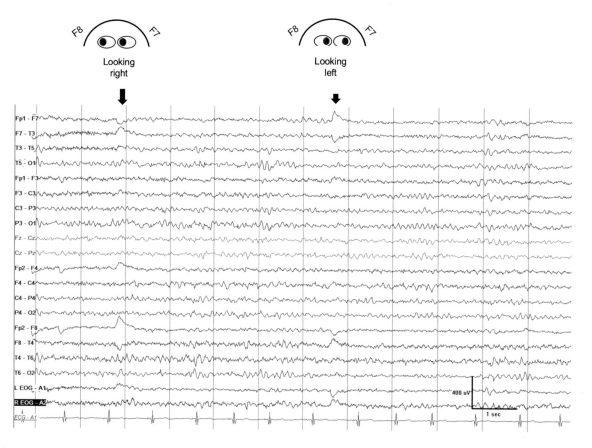

Figure 2.8 Lateral eye movement artifact. EEG showing artifact caused by lateral eye movement. This artifact is caused because the cornea is positively charged and it generates a positive potential toward the direction of eye gaze. Lateral eye movement is recorded mostly by F7 and F8 electrodes.

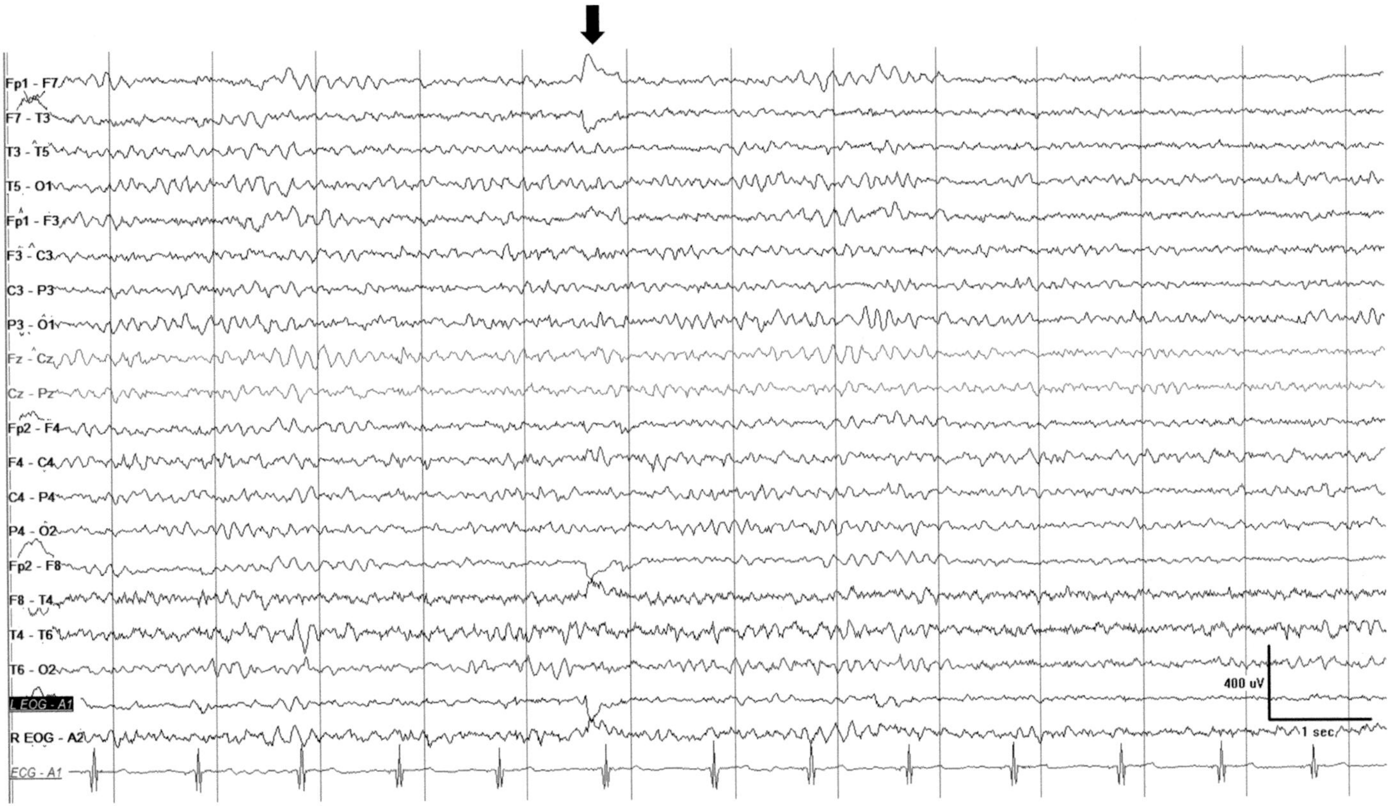

Figure 2.9 Lateral eye movement artifact. EEG showing positive potential in F7 and negative potential in F8 electrode (in this case, the patient is looking to the left [arrow]). Also note a small lateral rectus spike in F7. This artifact is caused because the cornea is positively charged and it generates a positive potential toward the direction of eye gaze.

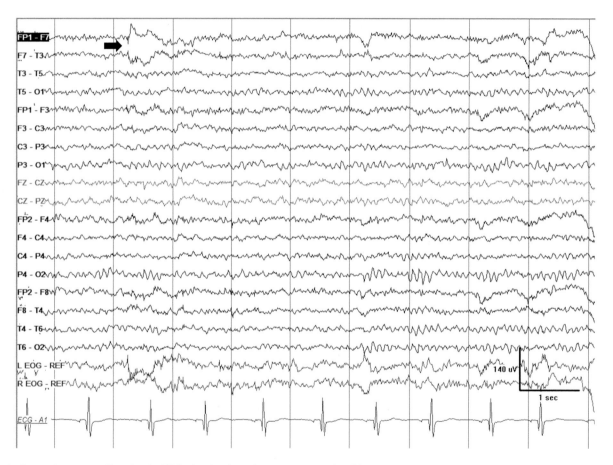

Figure 2.10   Lateral rectus spike. Awake EEG showing lateral eye movement (positive potential in F7) preceded by a high-amplitude spike (arrow) that corresponds to the EMG spike recorded during the lateral rectus muscle contraction.

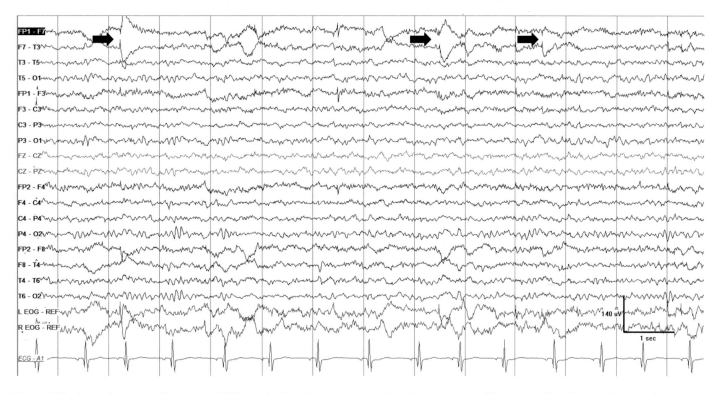

Figure 2.11   Lateral rectus spike. Awake EEG showing lateral eye movement (positive potential in F7) preceded by a high-amplitude spike (arrows) that correspond to the EMG spike recorded during the lateral rectus muscle contraction. (Courtesy: Kevin McGinnis.)

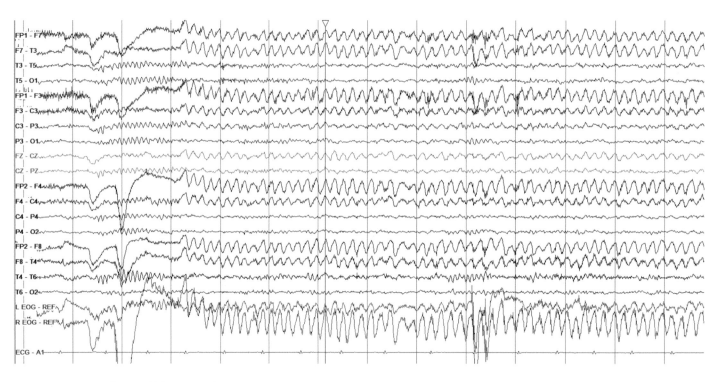

Figure 2.12   Eyelid flutter. EEG showing frontal 5 Hz monomorphic, high-amplitude theta waves associated with eyelid flutter.

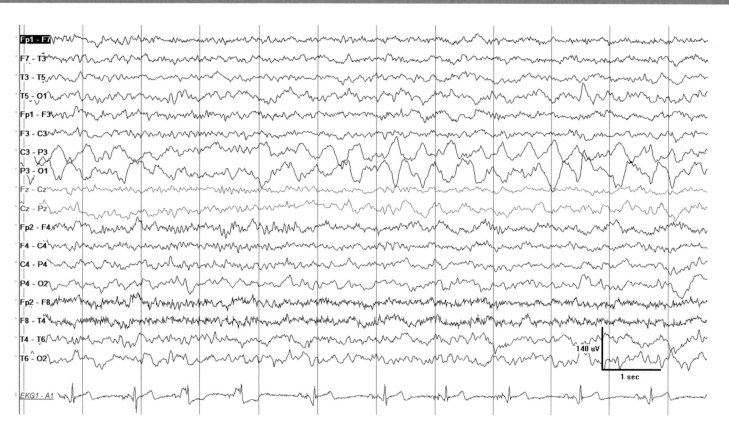

Figure 2.13 Electrode artifact. EEG showing electrode (P3) artifact on the 7th and 8th channels. This type of artifact is easily corrected by the technician by removing the electrode, cleaning the skin, and reapplying the collodion and electrode. (Courtesy: Ashley Kooney.)

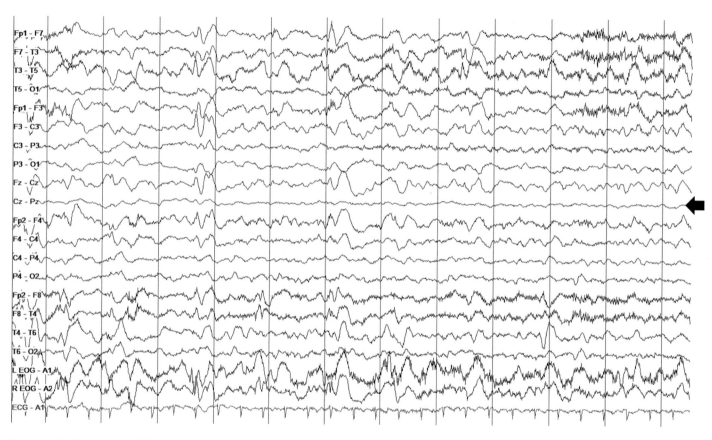

Figure 2.14   Salt bridge. EEG showing a salt bridge between Cz and Pz, characterized by low-amplitude recording (arrow).

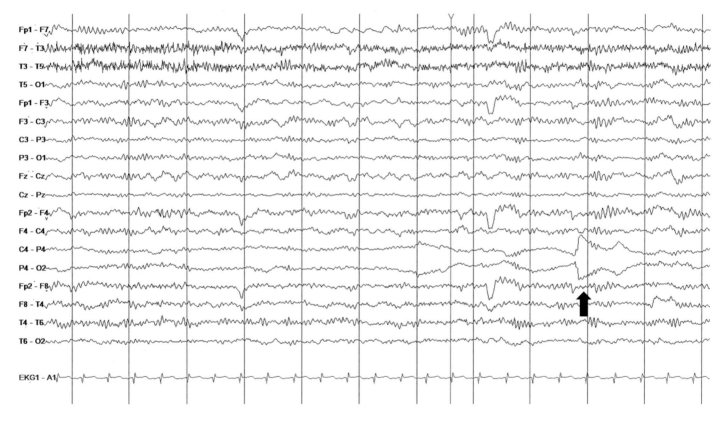

Figure 2.15 Electrode "pop." EEG showing electrode (P4) "pop." The artifact morphology characterized by a step component followed by a gradual return to the baseline makes it easy to identify. This type of artifact is easily corrected by the technician by removing the electrode, cleaning the skin, and reapplying the collodion and electrode. (Courtesy: Jerry Velasquez.)

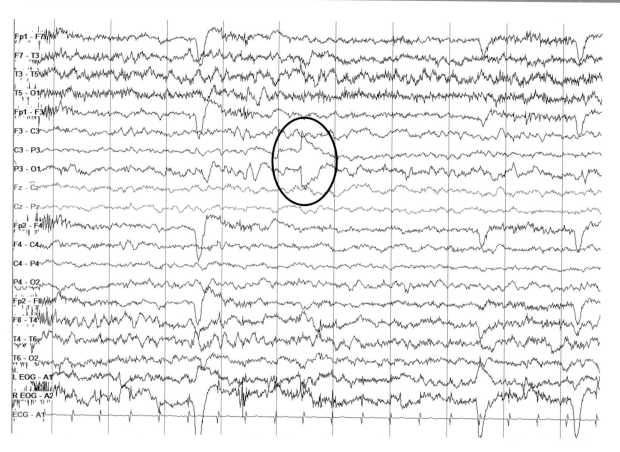

Figure 2.16 Electrode "pop." EEG showing electrode (P3) "pop." The artifact morphology characterized by a step component followed by a gradual return to the baseline makes it easy to identify it. This type of artifact is easily corrected by the technician by removing the electrode, cleaning the skin, and reapplying the collodion and electrode.

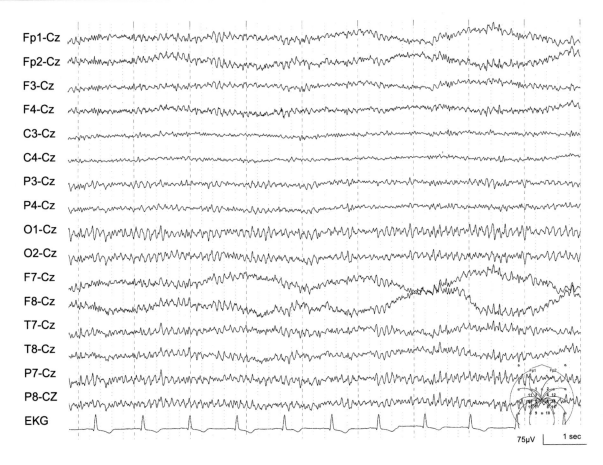

Figure 2.17   Sweat artifact. EEG showing sweat artifact, characterized by high-amplitude baseline oscillations in the frontal regions. It is caused by excessive sweat of the patient, which usually predominates in the forehead.

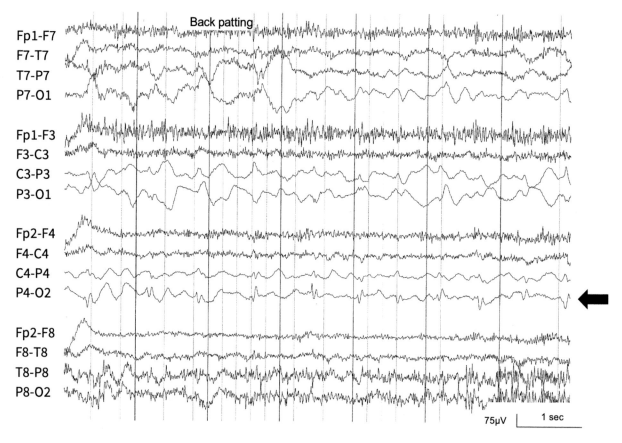

Figure 2.18   Electrode compression artifact. Rhythmic sharp waves in the 12th channel (arrow) caused by back patting to calm down this young patient. The technician identified this event during the recording, which is extremely helpful for those reading the EEG. The rhythmic characteristic of the artifact may suggest an epileptiform abnormality, or even a seizure, if not properly identified.

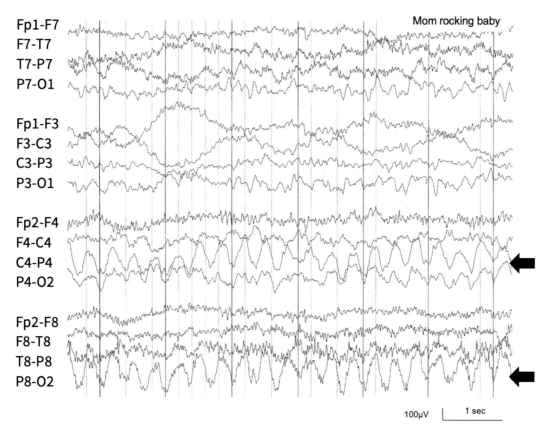

Figure 2.19 Electrode compression artifact. Rhythmic, sharply contoured slow waves in the posterior region of the right hemisphere (arrow) caused by the mom rocking the patient during the EEG recording. This artifact was caused by the rhythmic compression of the right posterior electrodes on the mother's arm. The technician identified this event during the recording, which is extremely helpful for those reading the EEG. The rhythmic characteristic of the artifact may suggest a seizure if not properly identified.

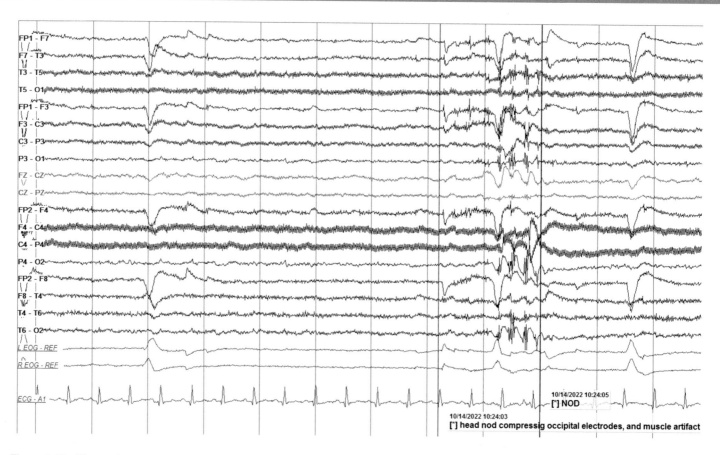

Figure 2.20 Electrode compression and muscle artifact. EEG showing artifact caused by the patient's head nod, which compressed the occipital electrodes (rhythmic slow waves). Also note diffuse spikes caused by muscle contraction and electrical current artifact (60 Hz) more prominent in the 3rd, 4th, 12th, and 13th channels.

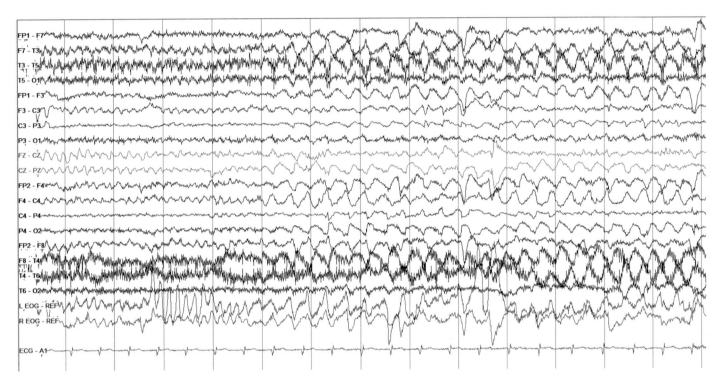

Figure 2.21 Rocking artifact. EEG showing high-amplitude rhythmic slow waves produced by the mother rocking the child to make him sleep.

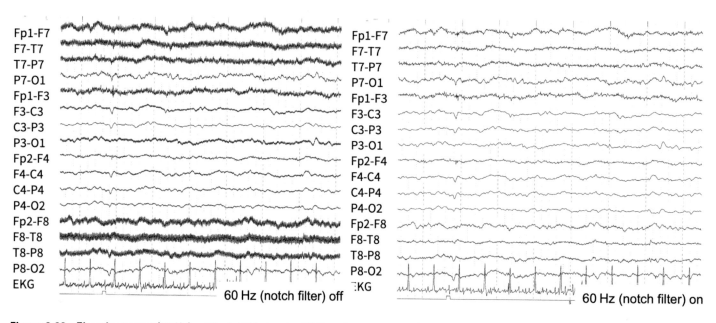

Figure 2.22   Electric current (60 Hz) artifact. EEG showing 60 Hz spikes most prominent at the frontal regions caused by electric current interference. Note that when the 60 Hz filter is on, there is great improvement of the artifact.

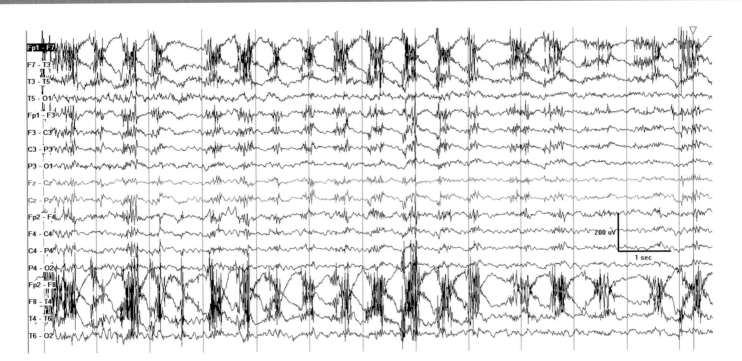

Figure 2.23   Chewing and glossokinetic artifact. EEG showing the patient chewing, which causes two types of artifacts: Rhythmic muscle artifact (high-amplitude and high-frequency spikes more prominent over the frontotemporal regions) and glossokinetic artifact. The tip of the tongue is negatively charged, and the base of the tongue is positively charged (which functions as a dipole). The tongue movement will cause rhythmic slow waves that are more prominent in the anterior electrodes.

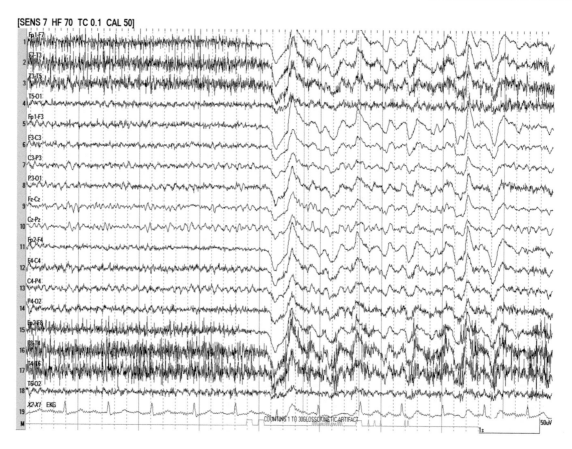

Figure 2.24   Glossokinetic artifact. EEG showing a glossokinetic artifact produced by counting out loud. The tip of the tongue is negatively charged, and the base of the tongue is positively charged (which functions as a dipole). The tongue movement will cause rhythmic slow waves that are more prominent in the anterior electrodes. (Courtesy: Marisha Hamid, R.EEGT, FASET.)

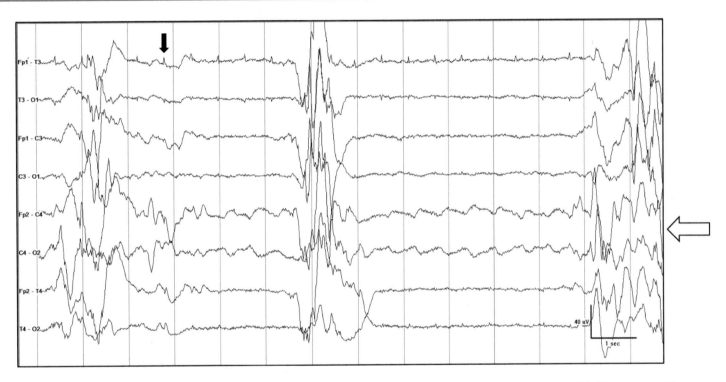

Figure 2.25 Pulsation artifact. EEG (8-channel bedside monitoring) showing burst suppression (sedation with pentobarbital) in a patient with severe head trauma. The patient underwent decompressive craniotomy (right side) and the C4 electrode recorded a brain pulsation artifact (white arrow). Also, note an EKG artifact (black arrow) over the left frontal region.

REFERENCES

Ebersole JS, Pedley TA. Current Practice of Clinical Electroencephalography. Philadelphia: Lippincott Williams and Wilkins; 2003.

Fisch BJ. Basic Principles of Digital and Analog EEG. 3rd Ed. Amsterdam: Elservier; 1999.

Hughes JR. EEG in Clinical Practice. 2nd Ed. Newton, MA: Butterworth-Heinemann; 1994.

Montenegro MA, Cendes F, Guerreiro MM, Guerreiro CAM. EEG na Pratica Clinica. Rio de Janeiro: Thieme-Reventer; 2022.

Tyner FS, Knott JR, Mayer WB. Fundamentals of EEG Technology. Volume 1: Basic Concepts and Methods. Philadelphia: Lippincott Williams and Wilkins; 1983.

CHAPTER 3

Activation procedures

Olivia Kim-McManus, MD

Maria Augusta Montenegro, MD, PhD

Activation procedures are used to increase the chances of recording epileptiform discharges in a routine EEG. The most common activation procedures are hyperventilation, intermittent photic stimulation, sleep deprivation, and sleep. The yield of activation procedures to trigger epileptiform abnormalities is higher for sleep and lower for hyperventilation and photic stimulation; and all three procedures are more effective to trigger epileptiform abnormalities in children than in adults (Baldin *et al.*, 2017). The most common epilepsy syndromes affected by activation procedures are shown in **Table 3.1**.

Table 3.1 Most common epilepsy syndromes affected by activation procedures

Hyperventilation	Intermittent photic stimulation	Sleep deprivation or sleep
Childhood absence epilepsy	Juvenile myoclonic epilepsy	Temporal lobe epilepsy
Juvenile absence epilepsy	Photosensitive occipital lobe epilepsy	Self-limited epilepsy with centrotemporal spikes
Focal epilepsy (focal intermittent slowing can be enhanced during hyperventilation)	Dravet syndrome	Developmental epilepsy with spike-wave activation on sleep
	Epilepsy with eyelid myoclonia	Juvenile myoclonic epilepsy (especially sleep deprivation)
	Neuronal ceroid lipofuscinosis	

DOI: 10.1201/b23339-3

HYPERVENTILATION

Hyperventilation should be performed in routine EEG for three to five minutes, followed by at least one additional minute of recording. Because hyperventilation depends on the patient's effort and may cause dizziness, the technician should encourage and reassure the patient during the procedure. Hyperventilation should be stopped immediately if the patient presents chest pain or if there is a change in the EKG rhythm (mild tachycardia may occur without further complications). Contraindications to hyperventilation include:

- Severe pulmonary disease.
- Moya-Moya disease.
- Severe carotid stenosis.
- Sickle cell anemia (or sickle cell trait).
- Pregnancy.
- Angina pectoris.
- Uncontrolled arterial hypertension.
- Hyperviscosity disorders.
- History of hemorrhagic or ischemic stroke, subarachnoid hemorrhage, or myocardial infarction in the past 12 months.

In childhood, adolescents, or young adults, hyperventilation can trigger bilateral and synchronous slowing, which can be exuberant (high-amplitude and delta frequency) in younger patients (**Figures 3.1–3.4**). In children, the slowing may predominate posteriorly and in adolescents, it is more prominent anteriorly (Fisch, 1991; Mendez & Brenner, 2006). Despite the anteroposterior predominance according to age group, the distribution of slow waves should be diffuse, without focal or persistent lateralization (**Figure 3.5**). One minute after the end of hyperventilation, slowing should disappear, with a return to previous baseline activity. Low blood glucose may exacerbate the slowing.

Hyperventilation is more effective to trigger abnormalities in patients with generalized epilepsies. Generalized 3 Hz spike-and-wave complexes are the most frequent epileptiform abnormality associated with hyperventilation (**Figures 3.6–3.8**). It may also trigger an absence seizure, and if it happens, hyperventilation should be stopped. Another frequent finding is focal slowing (or exacerbation of a previously noted interictal focal slowing), which may help localize possible epileptogenic regions (Holmes *et al.*, 2004).

INTERMITTENT PHOTIC STIMULATION

Intermittent photic stimulation should be performed during wakefulness using a strobe lamp 30 cm from the patient's eyes, at frequencies of 1, 3, 6, 9, 10, 15, 20, and 30 flashes/second, each performed in 10 seconds trains with a 10 second interval between each frequency. It should be performed with eyes open and closed, and the patient should be instructed to open and close his eyes a few times during the procedure. Photoparoxysmal response may occur immediately after eye closure (Panayiotopoulos, 1974). Due to the risk of triggering a generalized tonic-clonic seizure, the photic stimulation should

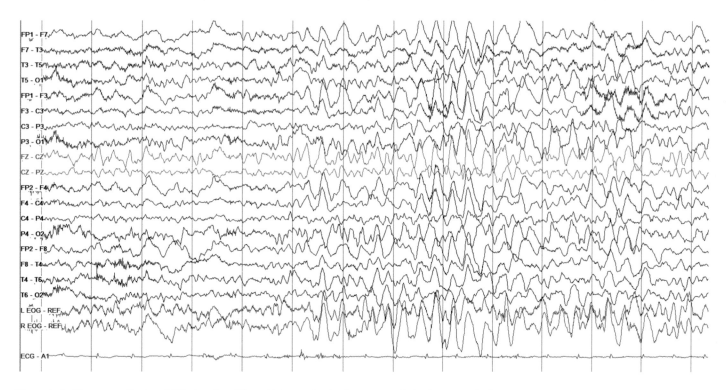

Figure 3.1 Hyperventilation. EEG showing diffuse high-amplitude slow waves during hyperventilation.

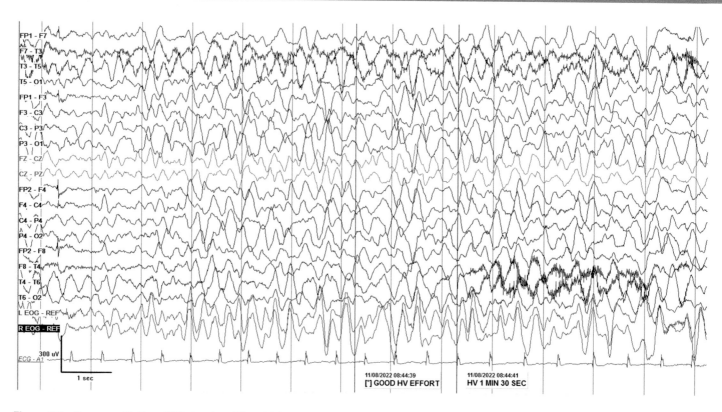

Figure 3.2   Hyperventilation. EEG showing diffuse high-amplitude slow waves during the first minute of hyperventilation.

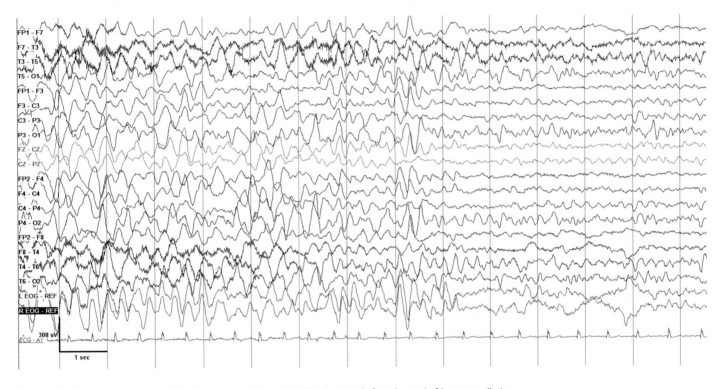

Figure 3.3   Hyperventilation. EEG showing return to normal background after the end of hyperventilation.

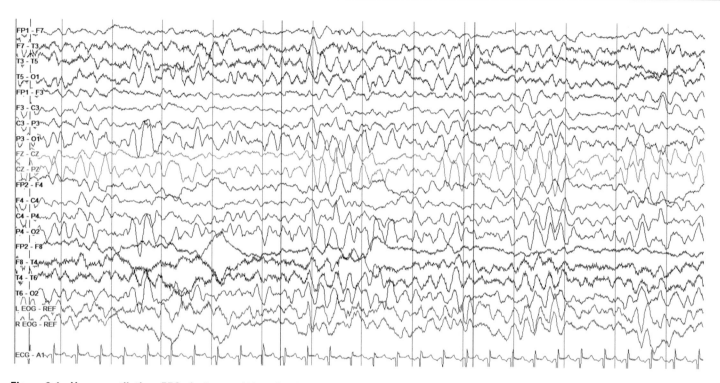

Figure 3.4 Hyperventilation. EEG of a 2-year-old boy showing high-amplitude slowing triggered by crying (which caused him to hyperventilate) during the EEG acquisition.

A

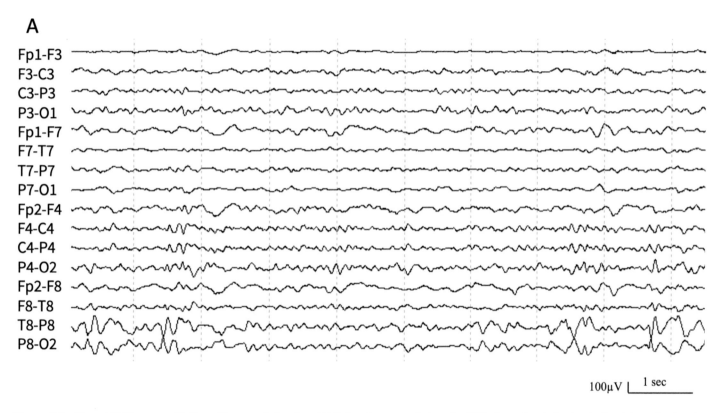

$100\mu V$ | 1 sec

Figure 3.5 (A and B) Hyperventilation: Abnormal slowing. (A) Before hyperventilation, the EEG shows focal slowing in the right parietal region seen in a child with focal epilepsy due to a structural brain lesion. (B) Same patient from A, now during hyperventilation. EEG shows diffuse slowing, more evident in the right hemisphere and in the parietal region. *(Continued)*

B

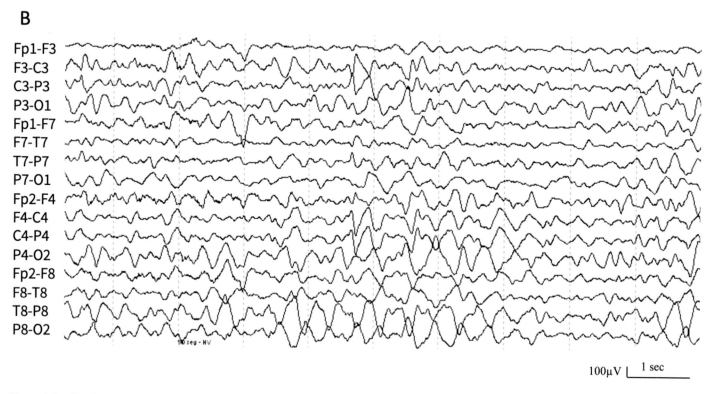

Fp1-F3
F3-C3
C3-P3
P3-O1
Fp1-F7
F7-T7
T7-P7
P7-O1
Fp2-F4
F4-C4
C4-P4
P4-O2
Fp2-F8
F8-T8
T8-P8
P8-O2

100μV 1 sec

Figure 3.5   *(Continued)*

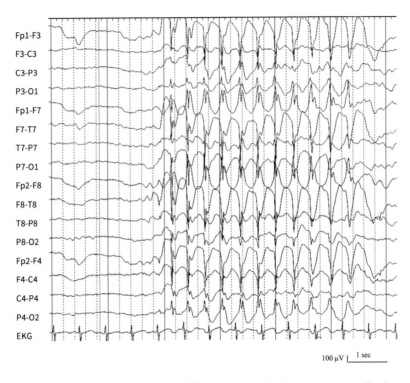

100 µV ⌊ 1 sec

Figure 3.6   Spike-wave complex triggered by hyperventilation. EEG of a 7-year-old girl showing generalized regular, 3 Hz spike-wave complexes triggered by hyperventilation.

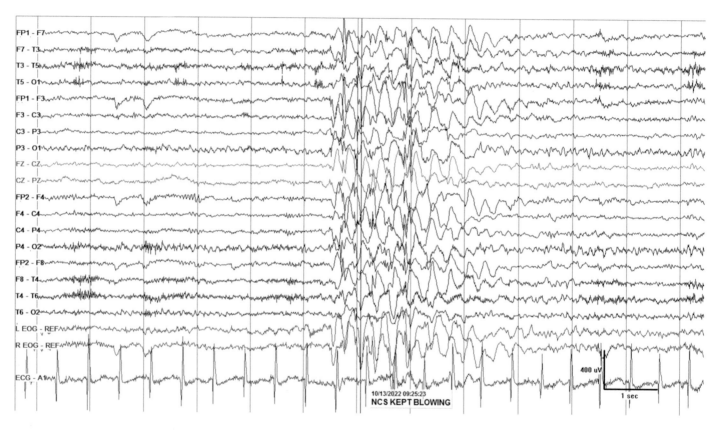

Figure 3.7 Hyperventilation. EEG showing generalized spike-wave complexes triggered by hyperventilation for less than 3 seconds. Not all discharges are associated with clinical signs (NCS: no clinical signs), especially if it has a short duration. Note that the patient kept blowing.

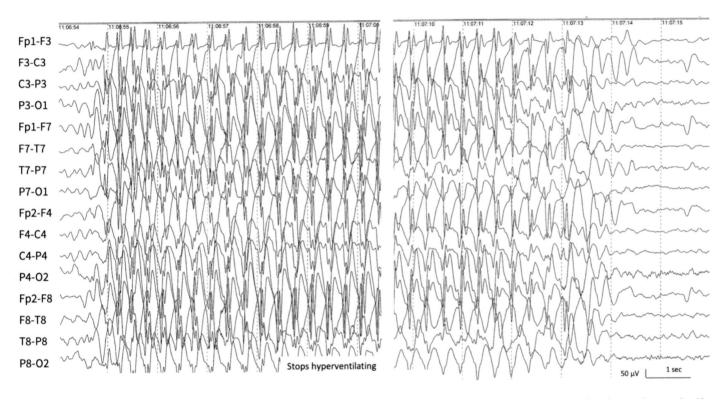

Figure 3.8   Absence seizure triggered by hyperventilation. EEG showing an absence seizure triggered by hyperventilation. It was characterized by the abrupt onset of generalized regular 3 Hz spike-wave complexes, with total duration of 17 seconds.

be stopped if a photoparoxysmal response occur. Three patterns of response might occur during intermittent photic stimulation (**Table 3.2**).

Photoparoxysmal response is more common at 14-18 Hz frequencies and it is usually generalized, but focal spikes or sharp waves may also be triggered. Occipital spike-and-wave or polyspike-slow-wave or posteriorly predominant generalized discharges may be triggered by intermittent photic stimulation in children with photosensitive occipital lobe epilepsy (Guerrini *et al.*, 1995).

Photosensitivity is more commonly associated with generalized epilepsies, especially juvenile myoclonic epilepsy, but it may disappear after the third decade of life (Jeavons *et al.*, 1986). It is important to note that some patients may have a photoparoxysmal response recorded on a routine EEG without ever presenting a seizure. Patients with neuronal ceroid lipofuscinosis may present high-amplitude occipital spikes during low-frequency intermittent photic stimulation (**Figures 3.9**–**3.16**).

Table 3.2 EEG response to intermittent photic stimulation

Photic driving	Registered on the parieto-occipital regions, and time-locked with intermittent photic stimulation (occurs with a delay of 70–150 ms). Its frequency must be identical or harmonic to the stimulus. It is an action potential of the visual system.	Normal phenomenon. POSTS and lambda waves are predictive of prominent photic driving response (Ebersole & Pedley, 2003).
Photomyoclonic response	Electromyography from eyelids and frontal scalp muscles, registered on frontal leads, they are time-locked to the stimulus. Associated with eye flutter.	Normal phenomenon.
Photoparoxysmal response	Epileptiform discharges triggered by intermittent photic stimulation. May outlast the stimulus by a few seconds.	Associated with photosensitive epilepsies (especially if it outlasts the stimulus).

SLEEP AND SLEEP DEPRIVATION

The frequency of epileptiform discharges often increases during sleep EEG, and several studies suggest that sleep deprivation may increase even more epileptiform discharges (**Figures 3.17** and **3.18**). Sleep deprivation acts as a stress on the central nervous system, done during wakefulness, especially in cases of idiopathic generalized epilepsy. Patients with temporal lobe epilepsy can benefit especially from tracing during sleep after deprivation (Degen, 1980).

If a patient diagnosed with epilepsy has a first normal routine EEG, sleep deprivation increases the yield of recording epileptiform discharges by 30% (Mattson *et al.*, 1965). However, there is no consensus on whether the waking or sleeping portion of the sleep-deprived EEG is most effective to activate epileptiform discharges (Méndez & Radtke, 2001; Pratt *et al.*, 1968).

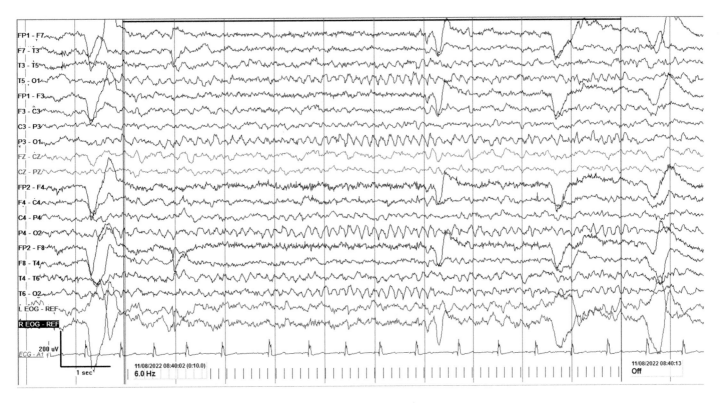

Figure 3.9   Photic driving. EEG showing rhythmic sharp waves in the posterior regions during 6 Hz intermittent photic stimulation. Note that it has the same frequency as the intermittent photic stimulation.

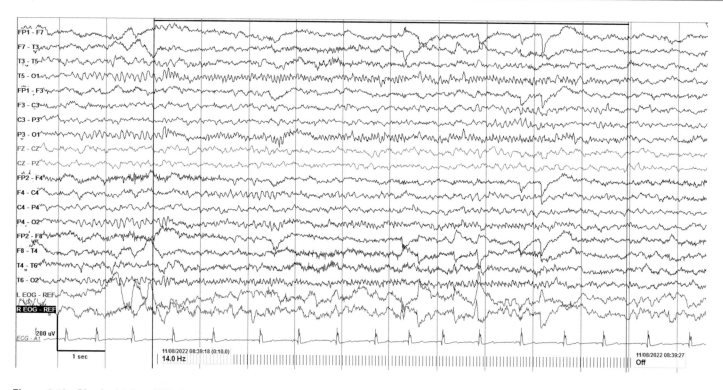

Figure 3.10   Photic driving. EEG showing rhythmic sharp waves in the posterior regions during 14 Hz intermittent photic stimulation. Note that it has the same frequency as the intermittent photic stimulation.

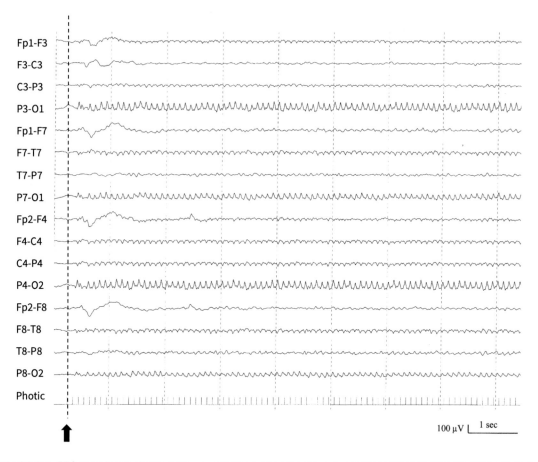

Figure 3.11   Photic driving. EEG showing rhythmic sharp waves in the posterior regions during intermittent photic stimulation. Note that it has the exact same frequency as the intermittent photic stimulation, but because it is an evoked potential, it starts a few milliseconds after the first photic flash (arrow).

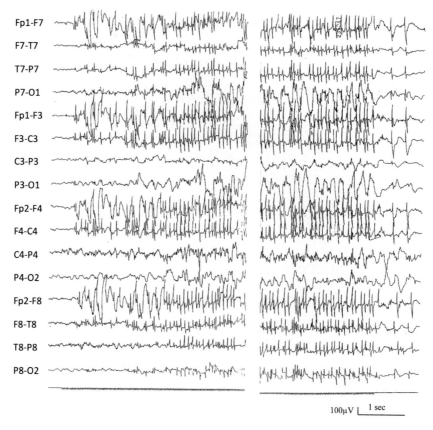

Figure 3.12   Photomyoclonic response. EEG showing high-amplitude spikes (muscle artifacts) in the frontal regions during the intermittent photic stimulation. (Reproduced with permission from Montenegro *et al.*, 2022.)

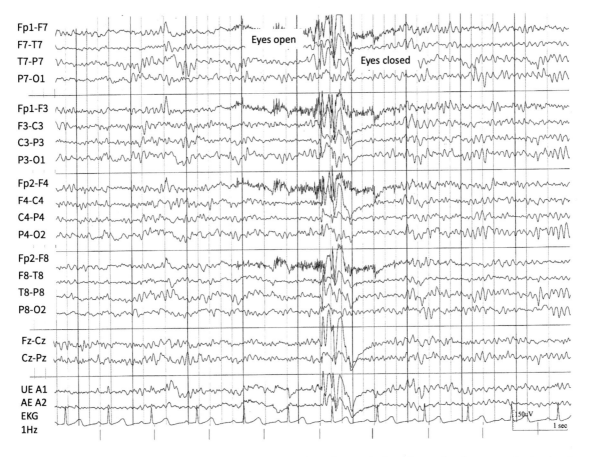

Figure 3.13 Photoparoxysmal response. EEG of a 15-year-old girl with juvenile myoclonic epilepsy showing generalized polyspike-wave during intermittent photic stimulation.

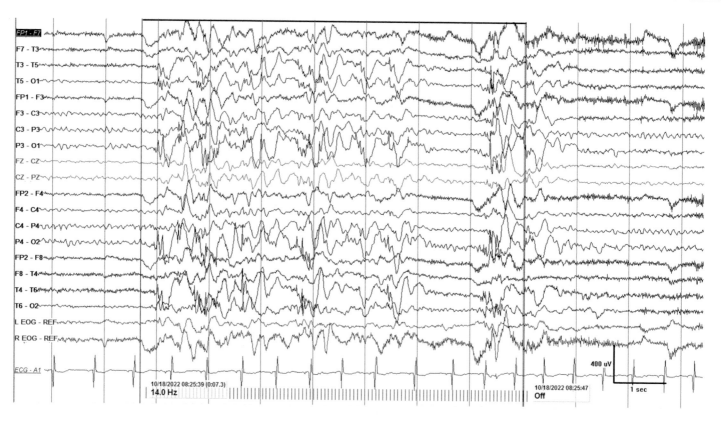

Figure 3.14   Photoparoxysmal response. EEG showing photoparoxysmal response during 14 Hz intermittent photic stimulation, characterized by generalized irregular spike-wave complexes.

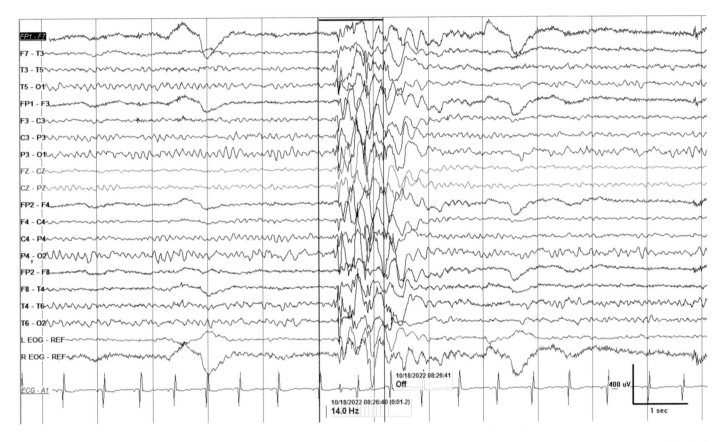

Figure 3.15   Photoparoxysmal response. EEG from the same patient showing generalized irregular spike-wave complexes when the 14 Hz photic stimulation was repeated. The photic stimulation was turned off after 1 second to prevent triggering a seizure.

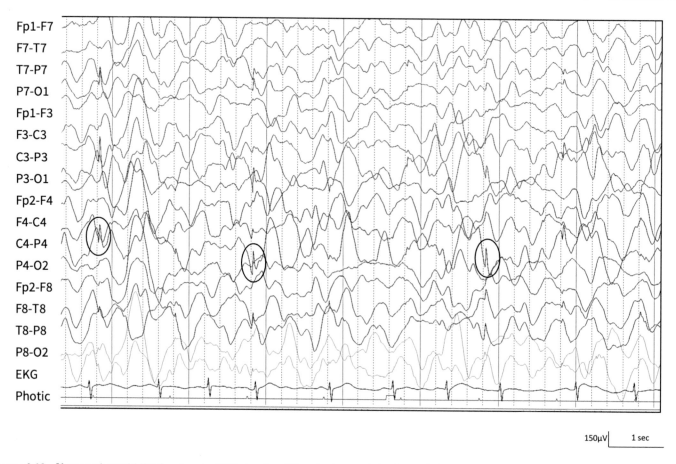

Figure 3.16   Neuronal ceroid lipofuscinosis. EEG showing diffuse background slowing and high-amplitude occipital spikes triggered by 1 Hz intermittent photic stimulation.

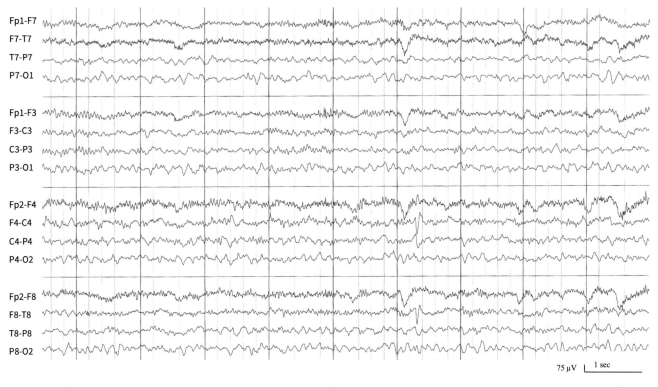

75 µV | 1 sec

Figure 3.17   Self-limited epilepsy with centrotemporal spikes (awake). EEG showing normal background and a single sharp wave in the central region (C4).

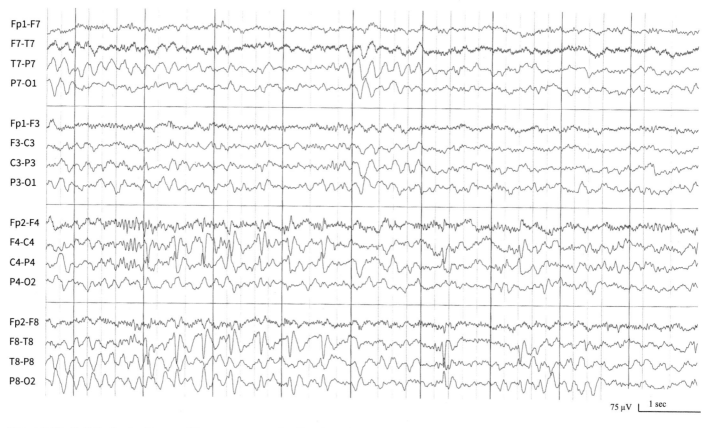

Figure 3.18   Self-limited epilepsy with centrotemporal spikes (sleep). EEG showing normal background during sleep and several sharp waves in the centrotemporal region. This is the same patient from **Figure 3.17**, same day of recording, note the sleep activation of the discharges.

In patients with focal epilepsy, interictal discharges are useful to lateralize the side of seizure onset. However, N1, N2, and N3 sleep stages might activate bilateral discharges, and it should be carefully evaluated to avoid false lateralization of the epileptic focus. The more reliable interictal discharges are often recorded during wakefulness and REM sleep, especially in patients with temporal lobe epilepsy due to hippocampal atrophy (Williamson *et al.*, 1993).

REFERENCES

Baldin E, Hauser WA, Buchhalter JE, Hesdorffer DC, Ottman R. Utility of EEG Activation Procedures in Epilepsy: A Population-Based Study. J Clin Neurophysiol 2017;34:512–19.

Degen R. A Study of the Diagnostic Value of Wake and Sleep EEGs after Sleep Deprivation in Epileptic Patients on Anticonvulsive Therapy. Electroencephalogr Clin Neurophysiol 1980;49:577–84.

Ebersole JS, Pedley TA. Current Practice of Clinical Electroencephalography. Philadelphia: Lippincot Williams & Wilkins; 2003.

Fisch BJ. Spehlmann's EEG Primer. 2nd Ed. Amsterdam: Elsevier; 1991.

Guerrini R, Dravet C, Genton P, Bureau M, Bonanni P, Ferrari AR, et al. Idiopathic Photosensitive Occipital Lobe Epilepsy. Epilepsia 1995;36:883–91.

Holmes MD, Dewaraja AS, Vanhatalo S. Does Hyperventilation Elicit Epileptic Seizures? Epilepsia 2004;45:618–20.

Jeavons PM, Bishop A, Harding GF. The Prognosis of Photosensitivity. Epilepsia 1986;27:569–75.

Mattson RH, Pratt KL, Calverley JR. Electroencephalograms of Epileptics Following Sleep Deprivation. Arch Neurol Chicago 1965;13:310–15.

Méndez M, Radtke RA. Interactions Between Sleep and Epilepsy. J Clin Neurophysiol 2001;18:106–27.

Mendez OE, Brenner RP. Increasing the Yield of EEG. J Clin Neurophysiol 2006;23:282–93.

Montenegro MA, Cendes F, Guerreiro MM, Guerreiro CAM. EEG na Pratica Clinica. Rio de Janeiro: Thieme-Revinter; 2022.

Panayiotopoulos CP. Effectiveness of Photic Stimulation on Various Eye-States in Photosensitive Epilepsy. J Neurol Sci 1974;23:165–73.

Pratt KL, Mattson RH, Weikers NJ, Williams R. EEG Activation of Epileptics Following Sleep Deprivation: A Prospective Study of 114 Cases. Electroencephalogr Clin Neurophysiol 1968;24:11–15.

Williamson PD, French JA, French VM, et al. Characteristics of Medial Temporal Lobe Epilepsy. II. Interictal and Ictal Scalp Electroencephalography, Neuropsychological Testing, Neuroimaging, Surgical Results, and Pathology. Ann Neurol 1993;34:781–87.

CHAPTER 4

Normal variants

Mark Nespeca, MD

Maria Augusta Montenegro, MD, PhD

Normal variants (also called benign variants) are normal physiologic discharges that have a sharp morphology that can cause their misinterpretation as being abnormal (interictal epileptiform discharges). They are relatively rare, usually occur during drowsiness or light sleep in young adults, and disappear with deep sleep (Kang & Krauss, 2019; Klass & Westmoreland, 1985; Stern, 2013). Although waveforms are often sharply contoured, normal variants have no clinical significance and are not associated with an increased risk of seizures.

It is not always easy to differentiate normal variants from true interictal epileptiform discharges and reading a highly abnormal EEG can be easier than reading a normal recording that has a normal variant. The misinterpretation of normal variants is not rare. Although an abnormal EEG is not enough to establish the diagnosis of epilepsy, it can be associated with loss of driving privileges, employment restrictions, and unnecessary exposure to antiseizure medication (Kang & Krauss, 2019; Tatum, 2013).

Interictal epileptiform discharges usually are clearly distinguishable from the normal background. Most are characterized by a surface-negative wave with sharp morphology often, but not necessarily, followed by a slow wave. In addition, the angle of the upward deflection is different from the angle of the downward deflection (**Figure 4.1**; IFSECN, 1974). Epileptogenic discharges usually display an electrical field identified on adjacent electrodes; however, non-epileptogenic potentials may also have a field evident in adjacent electrodes.

DOI: 10.1201/b23339-4

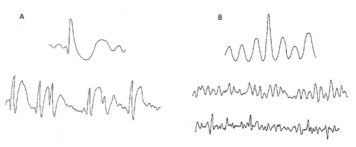

Figure 4.1   Difference of (A) epileptiform and (B) non-epileptiform discharges. Epileptiform discharges usually are clearly distinguishable from the normal background, are surface-negative, and follow a slow wave, with an upward deflection different from the angle of the downward deflection.

The most common normal variants are described below:

6 Hz Spike-and-Wave (Phantom Spike and Wave)

- Age: Adolescents and young adults.
- Localization: Diffuse.
- Frequency: 4–7 Hz (mainly 6 Hz).
- Duration: 1–2 seconds.
- When it occurs: Awake or N1 sleep.
- Characteristics: Bursts of low amplitude (<40 µV) 6 Hz (5–7 Hz) slow waves preceded by a very small spike (phantom spike); the slow wave is more prominent and occur in bursts of 3-4 seconds (**Figure 4.2**). There are two types: FOLD (female, occipital, lower amplitude, drowsiness) and WHAM (wake, high-amplitude, anterior, male).

14-and-6 Hz Positive Bursts

- Age: Children, adolescents, and young adults.
- Localization: Temporal (unilateral or bilateral).
- Frequency: 5–7 Hz and 13–17 Hz.
- Duration: Less than 2 seconds.
- When it occurs: N1 or N2 sleep.
- Characteristics: Bursts (1–2 seconds) of arciform spikes (round 14 Hz) and slow waves (around 6 Hz), more commonly seen in the temporal regions, with broad distribution, manifested with broad regional positivity maximal in the temporoparietal region. May have mixed frequencies as described above. May be fragmented and of only 200–500 ms duration. Best seen in ipsilateral ear referential and common average montages (**Figures 4.3–4.6**).

Alpha Variant

- Age: Older children, adolescents, adults (any age).
- Localization: Occipital.
- Frequency: Infra or supra-harmonic (slow alpha, fast alpha).
- Duration: 3–4 seconds.
- When it occurs: Wakefulness.

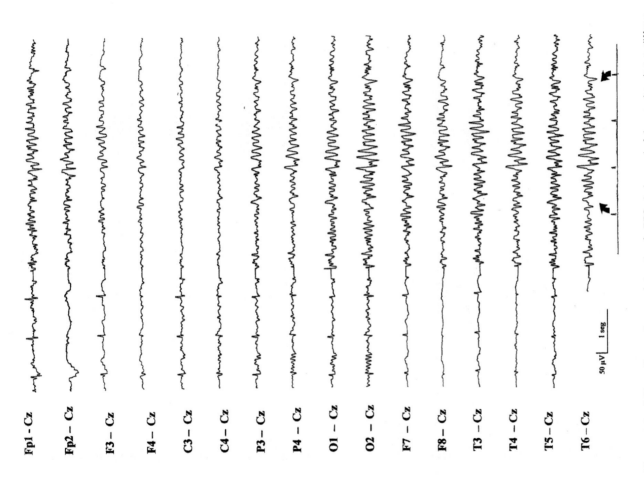

Figure 4.2 6 Hz spike-and-wave (phantom). EEG during wakefulness showing a diffuse burst of 6 Hz waves for 3 seconds (arrows) (Reproduced with permission from Montenegro et al., 2022.)

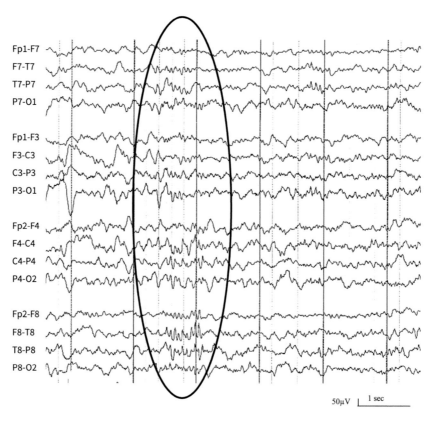

Figure 4.3   14-and-6 positive spikes. EEG showing a train of spikes and sharp waves more evident in the temporal regions.

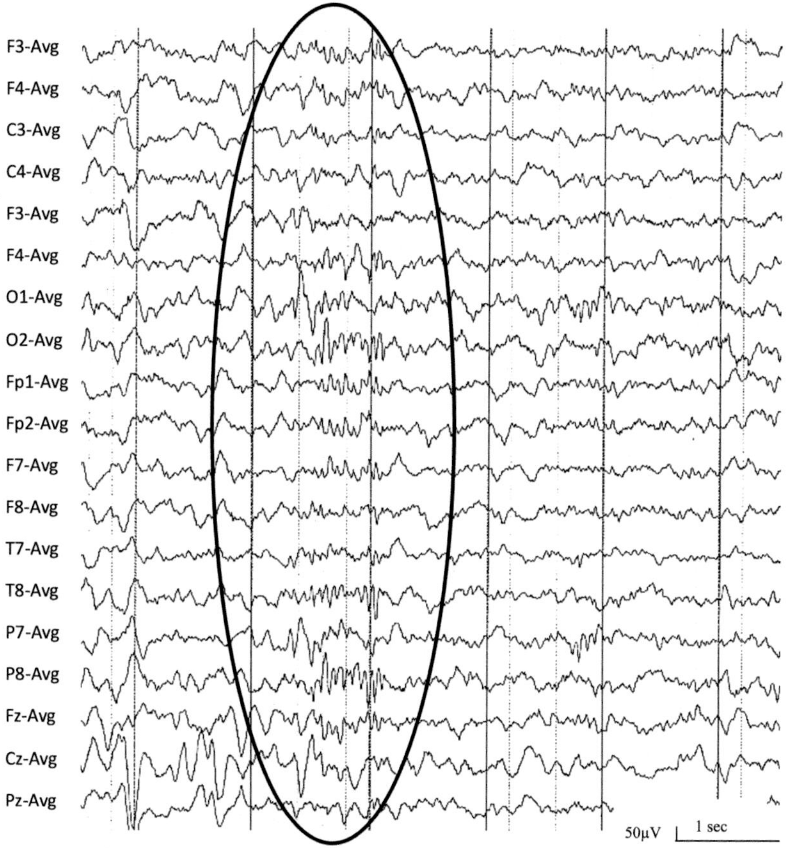

Figure 4.4   14-and-6 positive spikes. This is the same EEG moment from the previous figure, now at a referential montage. It shows a train of spikes with sharp morphology.

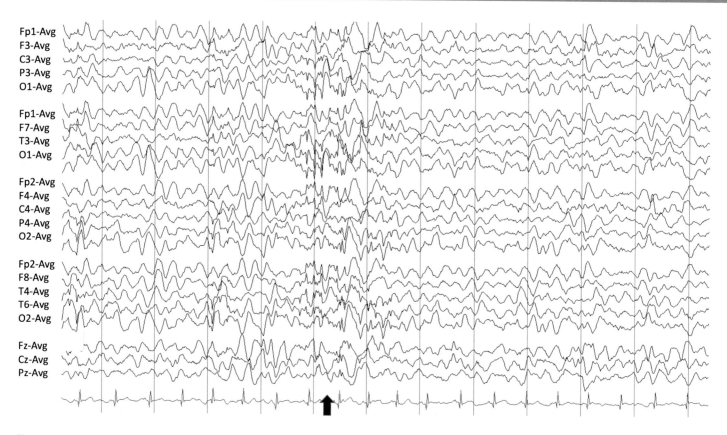

Figure 4.5   14-and-6 positive spikes. EEG showing a run of spikes (arrow) and sharp waves more evident in the temporal regions.

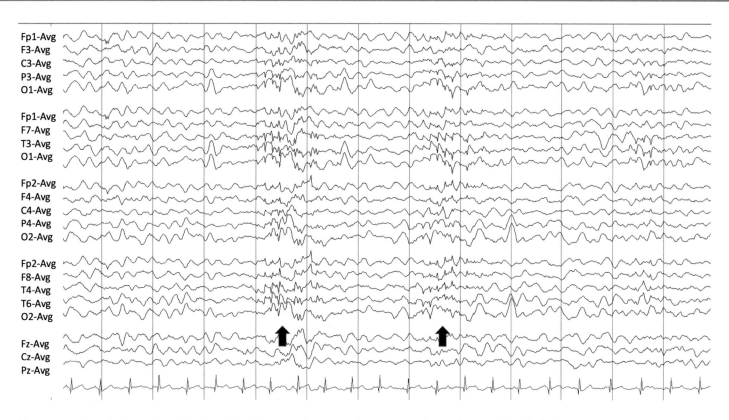

Figure 4.6 14-and-6 positive spikes. EEG showing a run of spikes and sharp waves (arrows) more evident in the temporal regions.

- Characteristics: Rhythmic, sinusoidal (fast alpha has a spike-like morphology), slow waves with notched appearance (summation of one or two waves). It must have a harmonic frequency of the patient's posterior dominant rhythm and is reactive to eye-opening (**Figures 4.7** and **4.8**).

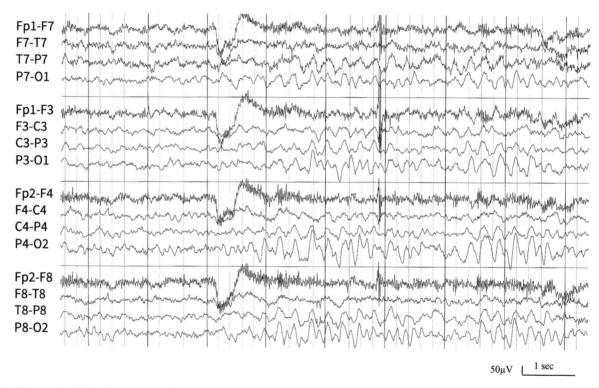

50µV ⌊ 1 sec

Figure 4.7   Alpha variant (slow). EEG showing alpha variant slower than the baseline posterior dominant rhythm frequency (after eye closure) in the occipital regions. It occurs in any age during wakefulness.

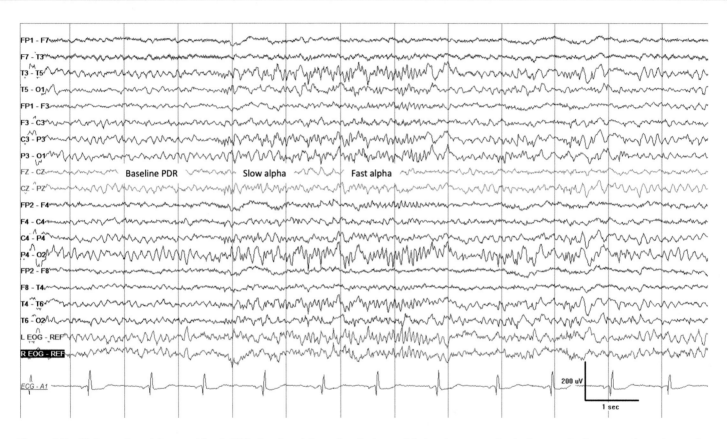

Figure 4.8   Alpha variant (slow and fast). EEG showing alpha variant in the occipital regions, note that it changes the frequency from slow to fast harmonic.

BETS, Small Sharp Spikes, Benign Sporadic Sleep Spikes

- Age: Adults (extremely rare in pre-adolescent children).
- Localization: Broad field usually temporal, with distribution to frontal; unilateral or bilateral (may be synchronous or asynchronous).
- Duration: Waveform is less than <50 ms, usually isolated, and not in repetitive trains; may occur several in a sequence but with an interval of several seconds between each spike.
- When it occurs: N1 or N2 sleep.
- Characteristics: Low amplitude (usually <50 μV) monophasic or simple diphasic morphology with steeply sloped second phase and broadly distributed in the frontotemporal region (**Figure 4.9**).

Breach Rhythm

- Age: Any age.
- Localization: Over or near a skull defect.
- Frequency: Increased amplitude and sharpness, especially faster frequencies.
- Duration: Continuous.
- When it occurs: Wakefulness, drowsiness, or sleep.
- Characteristics: Higher voltage amplitude of the background activity captured over a skull defect (**Figure 4.10**).

Frontal Arousal Rhythms in Children

- Age: Childhood.
- Localization: Bilateral frontal regions, but can be diffuse.
- Frequency: 7–10 Hz monomorphic.
- When it occurs: Arousal.
- Characteristics: High-amplitude, symmetrical, rhythmic discharges for several seconds (**Figure 4.11**). May be sharply contoured.

Lambda

- Age: Children and teenagers.
- Localization: Occipital.
- Frequency: 4–5 Hz
- Duration: Runs of several seconds.
- When it occurs: Wakefulness.
- Characteristics: Positive sharp waves in the occipital region, seen with eyes open, during visual exploration; often has morphology of Greek letter lambda – λ (**Figure 4.12**).

Midline Theta Rhythm (Ciganek)

- Age: Adult, especially young adults.
- Localization: Central, usually maximum at Cz sometimes at Fz.
- Frequency: 5–7 Hz.
- Duration: Several seconds, as long as 20 seconds.

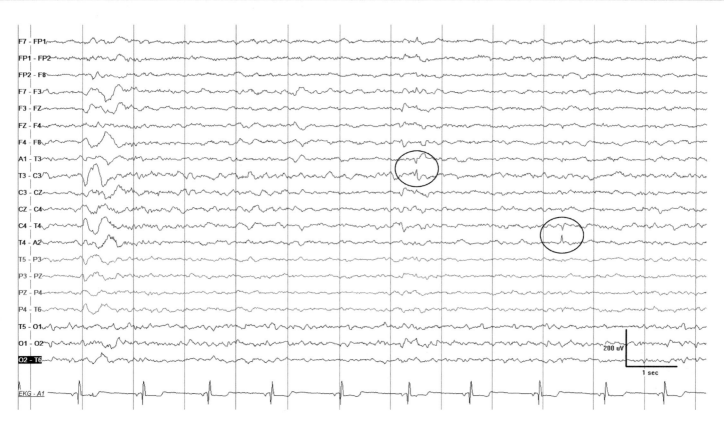

Figure 4.9 BETS, also called small sharp spikes. EEG during sleep of a 14-year-old girl showing low-amplitude spikes over the temporal regions.

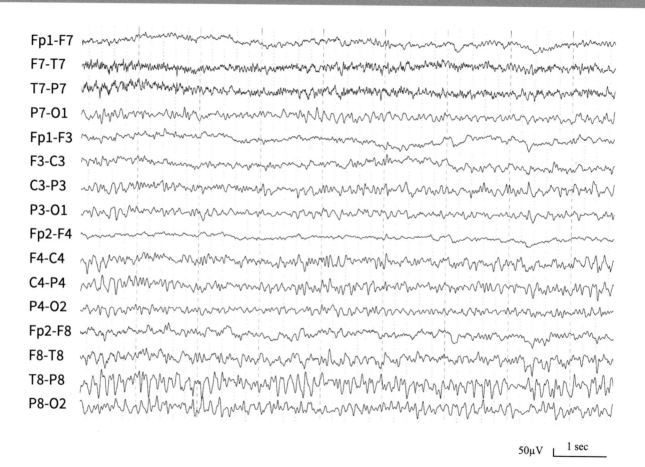

Figure 4.10   Breach rhythm. EEG of a patient with temporal lobe epilepsy that underwent epilepsy surgery. Note the increase in amplitude in right temporo-parietal region (under the skull defect).

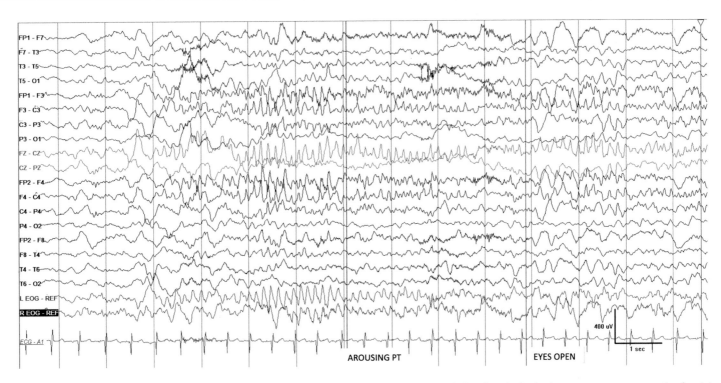

Figure 4.11   Frontal arousal rhythms in children. EEG of a 4-year-old boy during arousal showing rhythmic theta range waves over the frontal regions for several seconds.

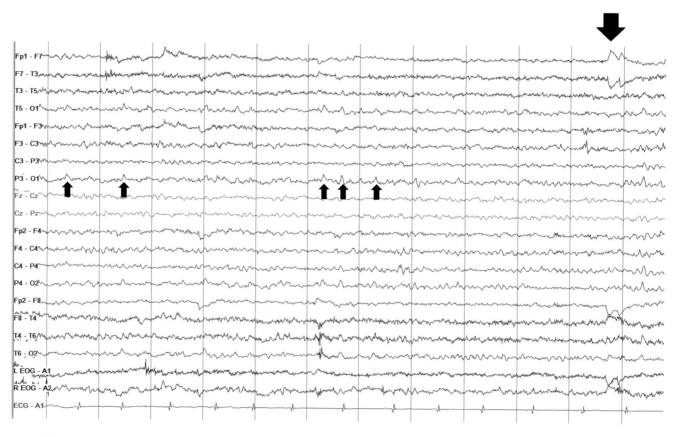

Figure 4.12   Lambda waves. EEG showing sharp waves in the occipital region (arrows) when the patient is awake with eyes opened (during visual exploration). Also note horizontal eye movement to the left (large arrow).

- When it occurs: Wakefulness or drowsiness. When only in awake state has been reported in patients with mesial frontal epilepsy.

- Characteristics: Midline theta rhythmic sinusoidal waves (it can be sharply contoured). It occurs in runs and may wax and wane. Usually, <50 μv amplitude. It has a higher prevalence in healthy controls (6%) *versus* patients (1%). Sometimes may distribute to adjacent parasagittal electrodes (**Figure 4.13**).

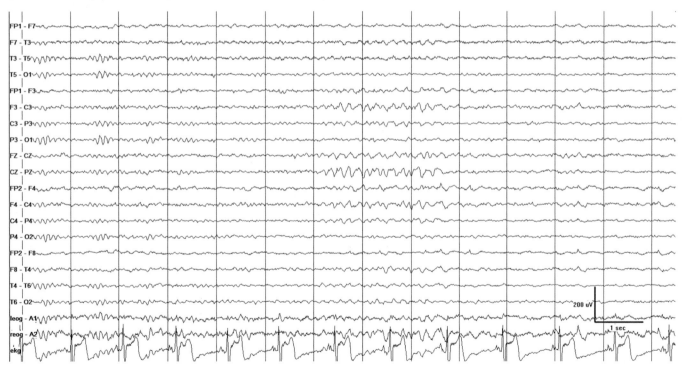

Figure 4.13 Midline theta rhythm (Ciganek). EEG during drowsiness showing rhythmic theta discharges in the central region.

Mitten

- Age: Children, adolescents, and adults.
- Localization: Frontocentral (best seen on referential montages [A1, A2]).
- Frequency: Around 2 Hz.
- Duration: Usually isolated, but may occur in runs.
- When it occurs: Non-REM sleep, especially with associated delta frequency background.
- Characteristics: High-amplitude sharply contoured v-wave, preceded by low-amplitude sharp wave (which may be formed by the last spindle), which produces the shape of a mitten. May be a variant of v-waves or K-complex (**Figures 4.14** and **4.15**).

Occipital Needle-Like Spikes

- Age: Children (congenital blindness), disappear in adulthood.
- Localization: Occipital (may be parietaloccipital).
- Frequency: Spike, <70 ms.
- Duration: Can be very frequent, even in runs.
- When it occurs: Wakefulness, or non-REM sleep.
- Characteristics: Medium- to high-amplitude spikes in the occipitoparietal region. May be activated by sleep. Often disappears in adulthood (**Figure 4.16**).

Positive Occipital Sharp Transient of Sleep (POSTS)

- Age: After the first decade of life.
- Localization: Occipital.
- Frequency: 4–5 Hz.
- Duration: Runs that can last several seconds.
- When it occurs: Non-REM sleep (more common in N1 sleep).
- Characteristics: Positive sharp waves in the occipital region (**Figure 4.17**).

Rhythmic Temporal Theta Discharges of Drowsiness

- Age: Adolescents (*teenagers*) and adults.
- Localization: Temporal, unilateral, or bilateral.
- Frequency: 5–7 Hz.
- Duration: Several seconds.
- When it occurs: Drowsiness.
- Characteristics: Rhythmic runs of sharply contoured theta waves in the temporal regions, which do not clearly evolve in amplitude, distribution, or morphology. Has also been described as "Psychomotor Variant" (**Figure 4.18**).

Subclinical Rhythmic Electrographic Discharge of Adults (SREDA)

- Age: Adults (usually older than 50 years-old), exceedingly rare in children and adolescents – per anecdotal reports.
- Localization: Temporal, parietal, may be asynchronous.
- Frequency: 5–7 Hz.
- Duration: Ranges from 10 seconds up to 5 minutes.

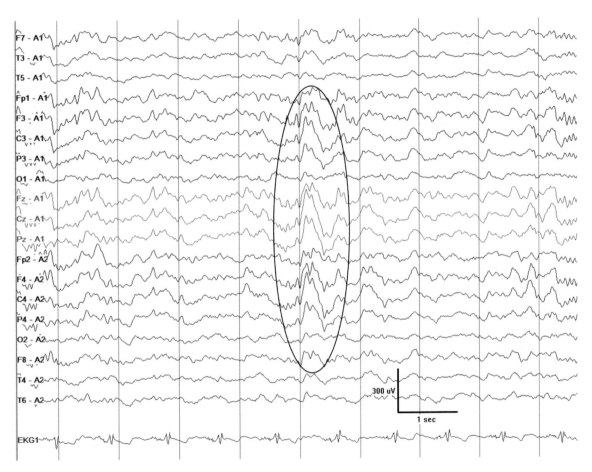

Figure 4.14   Mitten pattern. Sleep EEG showing sharply contoured high-amplitude wave preceded by a small spike of lower amplitude ("thumb of the mitten").

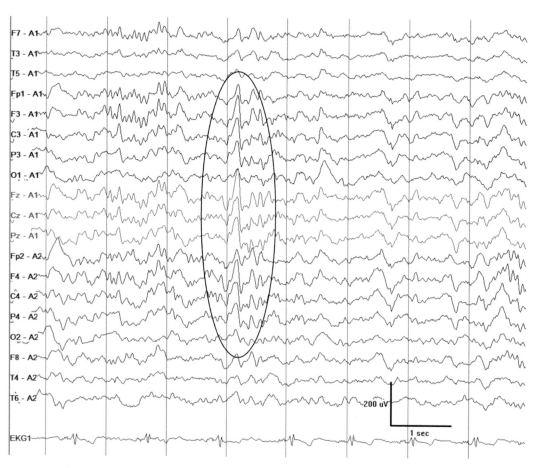

Figure 4.15   Mitten pattern. Sleep EEG showing sharply contoured high-amplitude wave preceded by a small spike of lower amplitude ("thumb of the mitten").

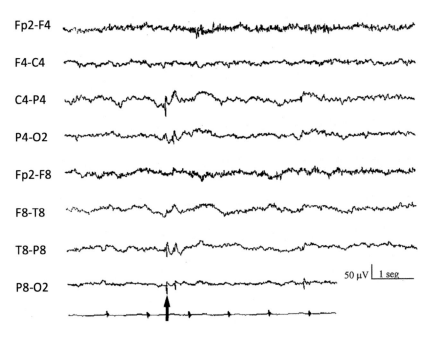

Figure 4.16   Needle like spikes. EEG of a child with congenital blindness showing occipital needle like spikes (arrow). (Reproduced with permission from Montenegro *et al.*, 2022.)

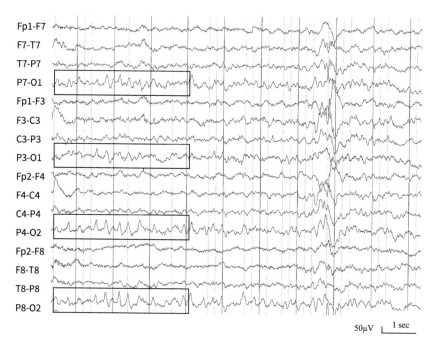

Figure 4.17   POSTS (positive occipital sharp transients of sleep). EEG showing a train of sharp waves in the occipital region during sleep (box).

- When it occurs: Wakefulness or N1 sleep, rare onset in N2 sleep.
- Characteristics: Abrupt onset of evolving delta rhythms of 40–100 mcv that then evolves into (diffuse burst) pattern of rhythmic sharply contoured 5–7 Hz waves lasting several seconds (up to 5 minutes). It is usually broadly distributed over posterior and parietal regions but may have a more focal distribution. May be precipitated by hyperventilation (**Figures 4.19** and **4.20**).

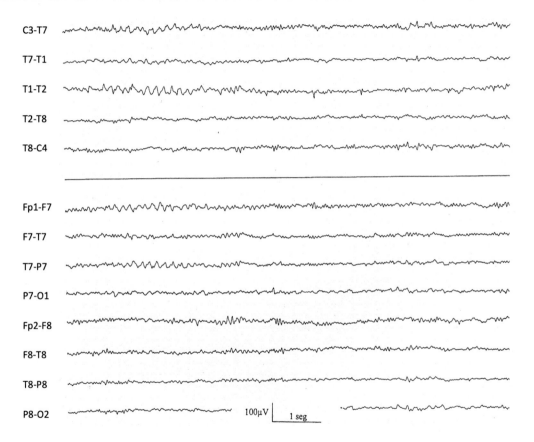

Figure 4.18 Rhythmic midtemporal theta discharges of drowsiness. EEG showing rhythmic theta waves in the left temporal region for 2 seconds. (Reproduced with permission from Montenegro *et al.*, 2022.)

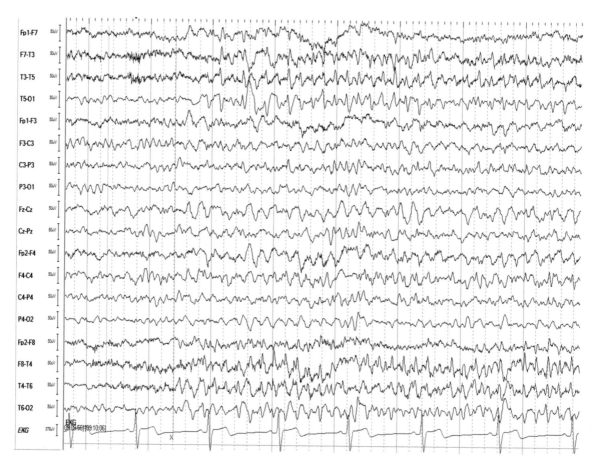

Figure 4.19   Subclinical rhythmic electrographic discharge of adults (SREDA). EEG showing abrupt onset of temporo-parieto-occipital sharply contoured rhythmic theta range waves for several seconds. (Courtesy: Marisha Hamid, R.EEGT, FASET.)

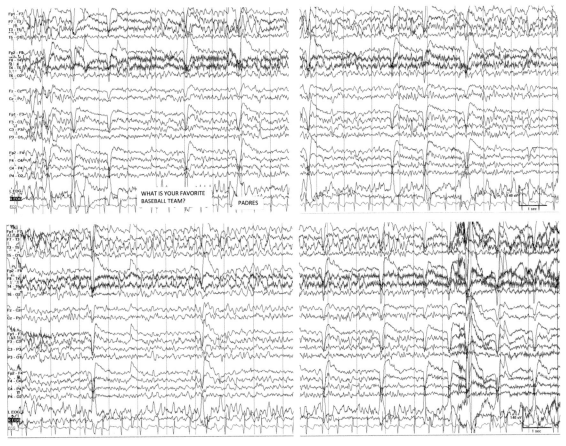

Figure 4.20 EEG of a 17-year-old boy during wakefulness showing rhythmic left temporal sharp waves in the theta range. Note that during the event, there is no impairment of awareness, as he is able to read, answer simple questions, and do simple math as well as normal naming and repetition. The rhythmic discharge lasts for several seconds.

Wicket Spikes, Wicket Rhythm

- Age: Adults.
- Localization: Anterior temporal and mid-temporal, unilateral, or bilateral.
- Frequency: 6–11 Hz.
- Duration: 1–3 seconds.
- When it occurs: Relaxed wakefulness or N1 sleep.
- Characteristics: Runs of repetitive monophasic sharply contoured waves, medium to high amplitude; when bilaterally synchronous may have shifting asymmetry (**Figure 4.21**).

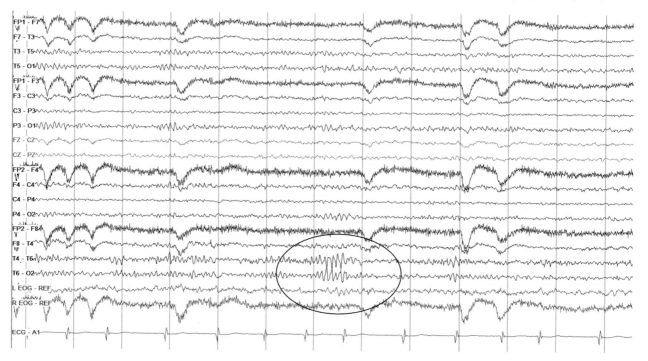

Figure 4.21   Wicket spikes. EEG showing sharp waves in the left temporal region. It usually has a frequency between 6 and 11 Hz, with arciform morphology, and is more common in adults during wakefulness and sleep.

REFERENCES

IFSECN. A Glossary of Terms Commonly Used by Clinical Electroencephalographers. Electroencephalogr Clin Neurophysiol 1974; 37:538–48.

Kang JY, Krauss GL. Normal Variants are Commonly Overread as Interictal Epileptiform Abnormalities. J Clin Neurophysiol 2019; 36:257–63.

Klass DW, Westmoreland BF. Nonepileptogenic Epileptiform Electroencephalographic Activity. Ann Neurol 1985;18:627–35.

Montenegro MA, Cendes F, Guerreiro MM, Guerreiro CAM. EEG na Pratica Clinica. Rio de Janeiro: Thieme-Reventer; 2022.

Stern JM. Atlas of EEG Patterns. Philadelphia: Lippincot Williams & Wilkins; 2013.

Tatum WO. Normal "Suspicious" EEG. Neurology 2013;80(Suppl1): S4–S11.

CHAPTER 5

Neonatal EEG

Jeffrey Gold, MD, PhD

Maria Augusta Montenegro, MD, PhD

The neonatal EEG is very different from the infant/child EEG, and weekly changes are seen continuously as the brain matures (**Figure 5.1**); therefore, the conceptional age (CA) is one of the most important variables for neonatal EEG interpretation. In addition, electrode placement can be different in newborns and many departments have their own established montages (**Table 5.1**). Although some institutions use all 21 electrodes from the 10–20 electrode placement system, due to the small head size seen in newborns, a reduced number of electrodes are suggested by the neonatal 10–20 neonatal electrode placement system (**Figure 5.2**).

The systematic evaluation of the neonatal EEG can be organized into four steps:

- **Step 1:** Establish if the background continuity is age appropriate.
- **Step 2:** Identify and establish if neonatal elements (beta-delta brushes, frontal waves/encoche frontales, temporal theta/alpha bursts, bifrontal delta activity) are age appropriate.
- **Step 3:** Identify sharp waves and establish if they are pathological (surface positive, occur in runs, frequency >1–2/minute).

DOI: 10.1201/b23339-5

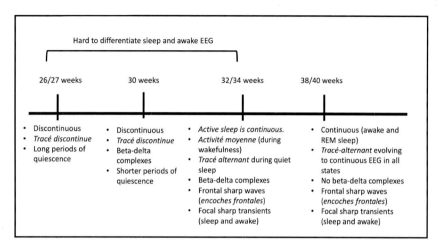

Figure 5.1   Maturation of the newborn EEG. Findings during the first weeks of life.

Table 5.1   Frequently used neonatal montages

FP1-T3	FP1-T3	FP1-C3
T3-O1	T3-O1 FP1-C3	C3-O1
FP2-T4	C3-O1	FP1-T3
T4-O2	Fz-Cz	T3-O1
FP1-C3	Cz-Pz	FP2-C4
C3-O1	FP2-C4	C4-O2
FP2-C4	C4-O2 FP2-T4	FP2-T4
C4-O2	T4-O2	T4-O2
T3-C3	T3-C3	T3-C3
C3-CZ	C3-CZ	C3-CZ
CZ-C4	CZ-C4	CZ-C4
C4-T4	C4-T4	C4-T4
FZ-CZ	EKG	EKG
CZ-PZ	Chest monitor	Chest monitor
EKG		
Chest monitor		

Source: Modified from Shellhaas *et al.,* (2011).

- **Step 4:** Identify possible seizures (rhythmic sharply contoured waves, may or may not evolve or have a surrounding field), if less than 10 seconds and without clinical symptoms it should be described as brief rhythmic discharge (BRD).

BACKGROUND

Until 32/34 weeks, the background is discontinuous, with long periods of quiescence (*tracé discontinue*). As the conceptional age increases, the periods of quiescence get shorter and the background becomes more continuous. Around 32/34 weeks, active sleep is continuous but quiet sleep still shows an "alternating" pattern of higher voltage discharges followed by brief lower voltage background (*tracé alternant*). In addition, around 34 weeks, wakefulness is characterized by a continuous admixture of delta and theta range waves (*activité moyenne*). The last stage to evolve into continuous discharges is quiet sleep, with *tracé alternant* evolving into continuous EEG until 42 weeks (Tsuchida *et al.,* 2013; **Tables 5.2** and **5.3**; **Figures 5.3–5.6**).

At 42/44 weeks of CA, the background should be continuous during wakefulness and sleep and characterized by an admixture of medium-amplitude theta and delta range waves. Dysmaturity is the persistence of EEG patterns that would be normal at younger

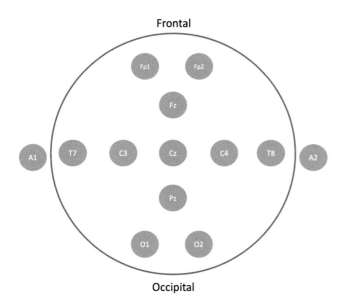

Figure 5.2   Neonatal 10–20 electrode placement. Note that fewer electrodes are used due to the small head size of most newborns.

Table 5.3   Normal neonatal background patterns

Normal neonatal background	Characteristics
Tracé discontinue	Short bursts of mixed-frequency high-amplitude waves (50–300 μV), followed by discontinuous (almost flat) pattern with long periods of quiescence. Quiescent periods are almost flat. Seen in premature babies. Period of quiescence gets shorter as the CA increases.
Activité moyenne	Wakefulness activity characterized by continuous mixed frequencies. It appears at about 34 weeks CA, as the quiescent periods of *tracé discontinue* get shorter until its complete disappearance.
Tracé alternant	4- to 10-second high-amplitude bursts (50–150 μV), followed by low-amplitude, mixed frequency activity. Seen at quiet sleep. Appears at 34 weeks CA. *Tracé alternant* evolves into continuous EEG near 42 weeks.

Note: CA: conceptional age; REM: rapid eye movement; NREM: non-rapid eye movement.

Table 5.2   EEG continuity according to age

Conceptional age	Awake	Active sleep	Quiet sleep
<32 weeks	*Tracé discontinue*	*Tracé discontinue*	*Tracé discontinue*
32–34 weeks	Continuous (*activité moyenne*)	Continuous[a]	*Tracé discontinue*
34–37 weeks	Continuous (*activité moyenne*)	Continuous	*Tracé alternant*
37–44 weeks	Continuous	Continuous	Continuous but with periods of *tracé alternant*

[a] Active sleep becomes continuous before the awake EEG shows continuous discharges.

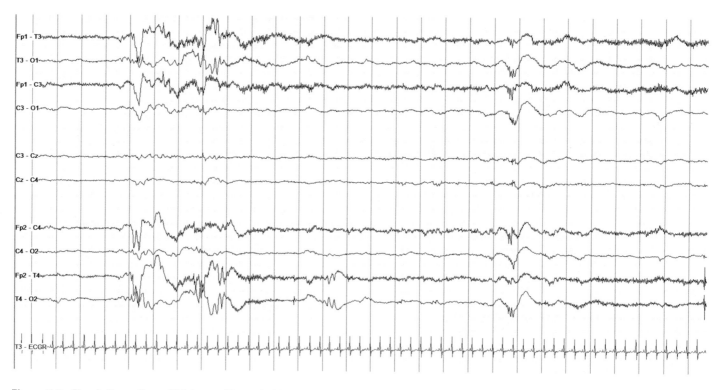

Figure 5.3   *Tracé discontinue*. EEG from a 28-week-old baby showing short bursts of slow and sharp activity followed by low-amplitude quiescent background.

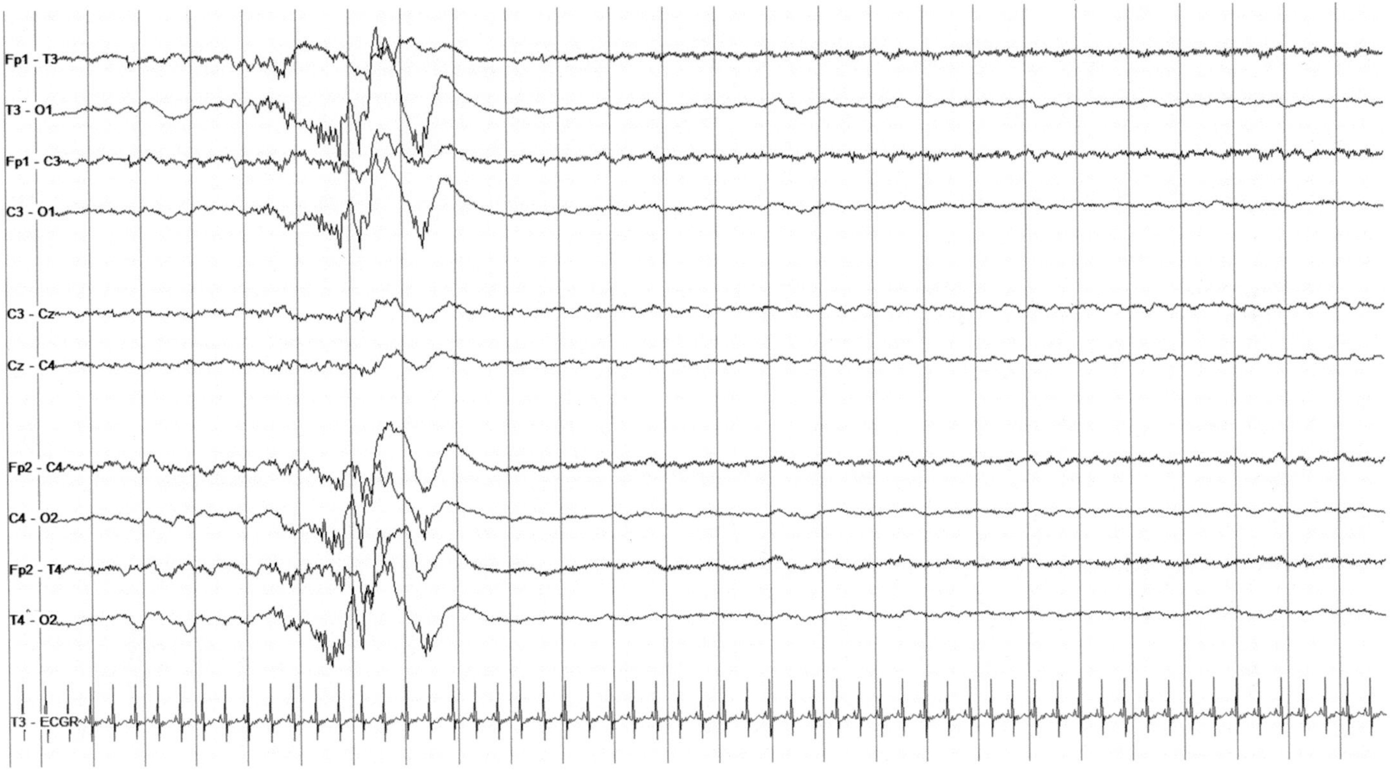

Fp1 - T3

T3 - O1

Fp1 - C3

C3 - O1

C3 - Cz

Cz - C4

Fp2 - C4

C4 - O2

Fp2 - T4

T4 - O2

T3 - ECGR

Figure 5.4 ***Tracé discontinue***. Another example of EEG from a 28-week-old baby showing short bursts of slow and sharp activity followed by low-amplitude quiescent background.

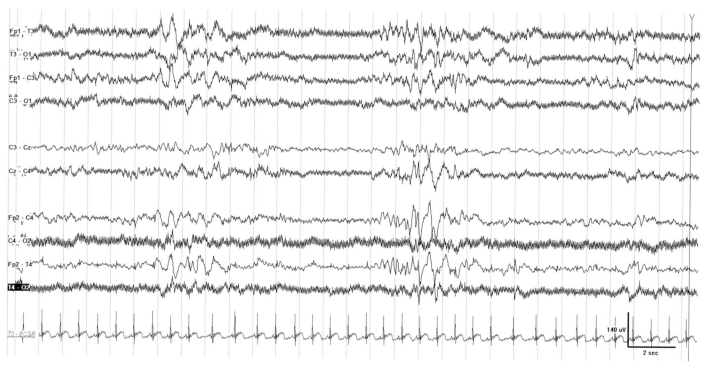

Figure 5.5 *Tracé alternant*. EEG during quiet sleep showing discontinuous periods of discontinuity during quiet sleep.

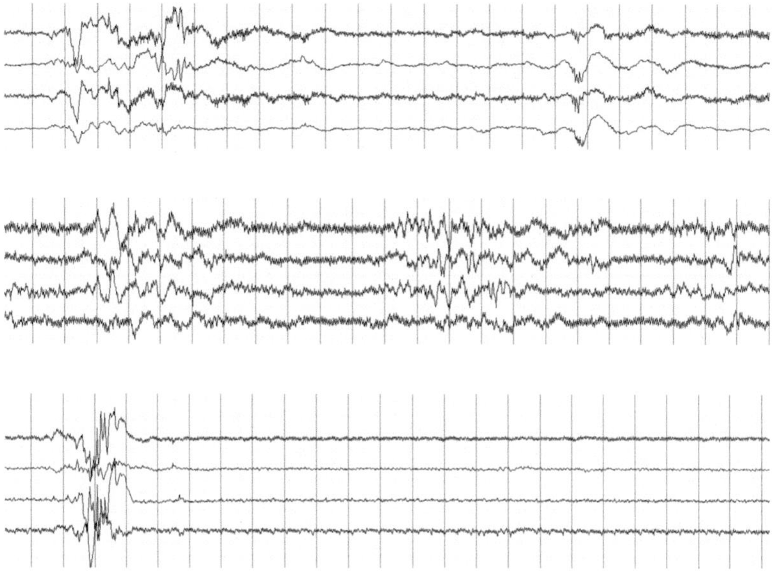

Tracé Discontinue
- Bursts: Admixture **of** frequencies
- Quiescence almost flat
- Premature

Tracé Alternant
- Shorter interburst interval
- Low voltage, but not as much as *tracé discontinue*
- 34 to 44 weeks

Burst-Suppression
- High-amplitude spike waves
- Suppression has very low amplitude
- Any age
- Critically ill neonate

Figure 5.6   Discontinuous patterns. Different characteristics between discontinuous patterns seen in the newborn period: *Tracé discontinue, tracé alternant*, burst-suppression.

gestational ages (excessive discontinuity, beta-delta complexes, etc.; **Table 5.4**; **Figure 5.7**).

NORMAL NEONATAL ELEMENTS

Once the background continuity has been evaluated, the electroencephalographer should look for normal elements that are seen in preterm and term newborns. The most common elements are sharp theta on the occipital of prematures (STOP), beta-delta complexes, frontal sharp waves (encoche frontales), bifrontal delta activity, and temporal theta and alpha bursts (**Figures 5.8–5.13**; **Table 5.5**).

Table 5.4 Awake and sleep EEG characteristics of background in the term newborn

Awake	Sleep			
	Active sleep	Quiet sleep	Transitional	Indeterminate
Continuous admixture of 25–50 µV theta and delta range waves (*activité moyenne*).	Continuous admixture of 25–50 µV theta and delta range waves.	*Tracé alternant* gradually evolves to continuous discharges until 42 weeks. It is replaced by 50–150 µV theta and delta range waves. Sleep spindles appear around 6 weeks of life.	Sleep stage between wakefulness, active sleep, and transitional sleep. It is a mixture of findings from both stages (the one that is ending and the one that is beginning).	Newborn has eyes closed but there is not enough information to establish the type of sleep.

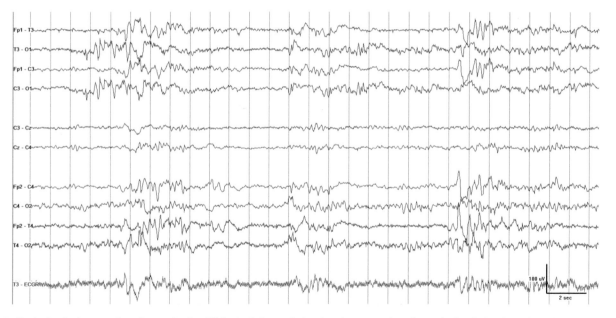

Figure 5.7 Pathological excessive discontinuity. EEG of a full-term baby showing excessive discontinuity during hypothermia.

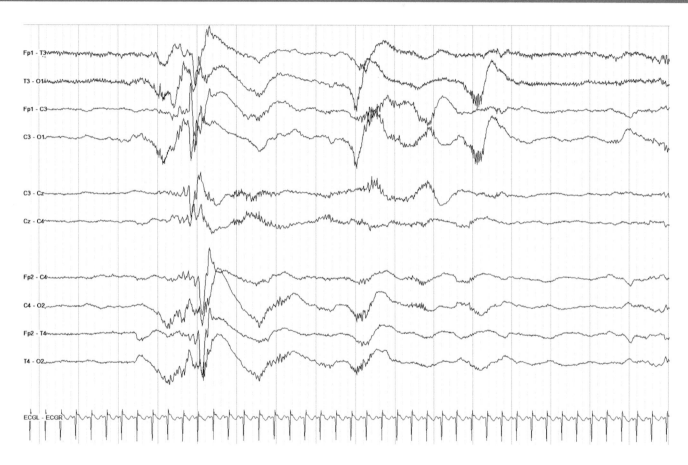

Figure 5.8 Beta-delta complexes. EEG of a 30-week-old baby showing beta-delta complexes characterized by fast activity with spindle-like morphology superimposed to a slow wave. Beta-delta complexes are seen in preterm babies.

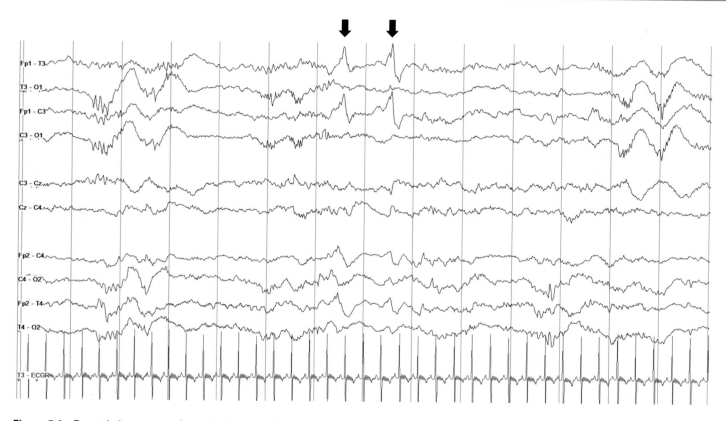

Figure 5.9   Frontal sharp waves (encoche frontales). EEG showing high-amplitude left frontal sharp waves with negative phase followed by positive phase (arrows). Also note beta-delta complexes in the 2nd and 3rd seconds and in the last seconds of the recording.

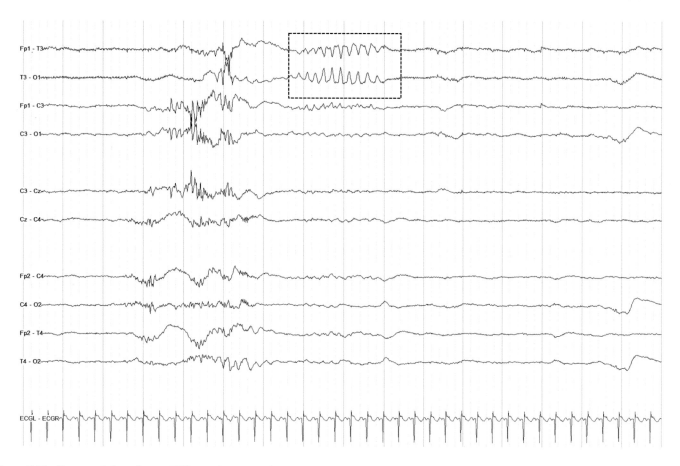

Figure 5.10   Temporal theta burst. EEG showing a run of theta range sharp waves with sawtooth appearance over the temporal region (box).

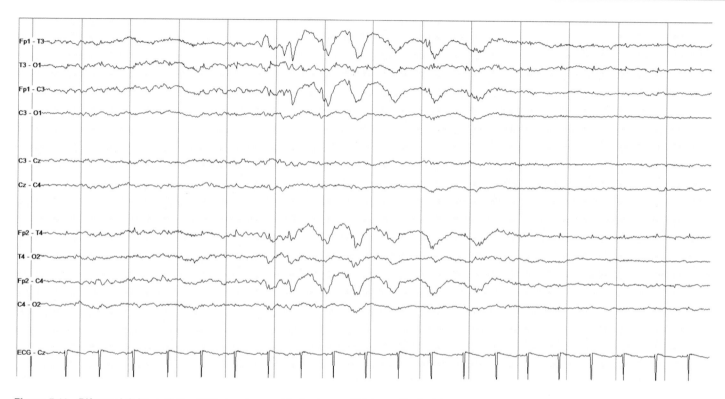

Figure 5.11   Bifrontal delta activity. EEG showing semirhythmic run of high-amplitude delta waves over the frontal regions. It was previously called anterior dysrhythmia, but the name was misleading because it is a normal finding.

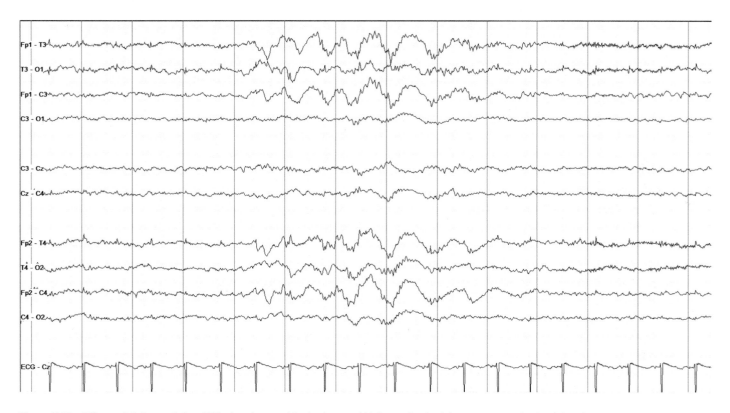

Figure 5.12   Bifrontal delta activity. EEG showing semirhythmic run of high-amplitude delta waves over the frontal regions.

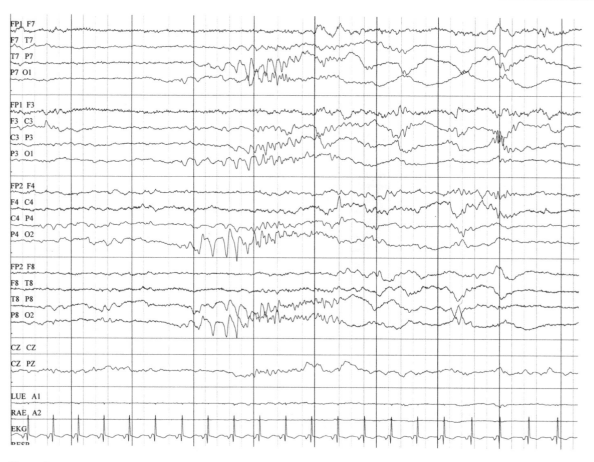

Figure 5.13   Sharp theta on the occipital of prematures (STOP). EEG showing bilateral occipital theta range waves over the occipital regions.

Table 5.5 Normal neonatal EEG elements

Normal neonatal EEG elements	Characteristics
Sharp theta on the occipital of prematures (STOP)	Occipital region (initially bilateral, but becomes unilateral as the newborn approaches 25 weeks). 22–25 weeks. 5–6 Hz discharge.
Beta-delta complexes (delta-brush)	First at central regions, later at occipital and temporal regions. 50–250 µV delta wave with superimposed fast activity. Hallmark of prematurity (26–38 weeks CA). 26–32 weeks: Mostly at REM sleep. >32 weeks: Mostly at NREM sleep. Should disappear after 38 weeks CA.
Frontal sharp waves (encoche frontales)	Frontal region (often bilateral). Single or in runs. Typical morphology is high-amplitude negative phase followed by positive phase. 34–44 weeks (peak 35 weeks CA). More frequent during transitional sleep. May occur in combination with bifrontal delta activity
Temporal theta bursts	Temporal region, unilateral. 4–6 Hz. 26–34 weeks (peak 30–32 weeks CA). Sawtooth appearance
Temporal alpha bursts	Temporal region, unilateral. 33 weeks. 1–2 seconds discharge in the alpha frequency, also with sawtooth appearance.
Bifrontal delta activity (previously called anterior dysrhythmia)	Frontal regions. Late pre-term to term weeks. Semirhythmic run of high-amplitude 1.5–2 Hz delta range waves over the frontal regions.

Note: CA: conceptional age.

ABNORMAL FINDINGS

Sharp waves are frequently seen during the neonatal period. Three main categories should be distinguished: Frontal sharp waves (encoche frontales, normal finding), physiological sharp transients (sharp activity with unknown significance, should not be considered pathologic; **Figure 5.14**), and pathological sharp transients (abnormal finding, **Figure 5.15** to **5.17**). The boundaries between physiological and pathological sharp

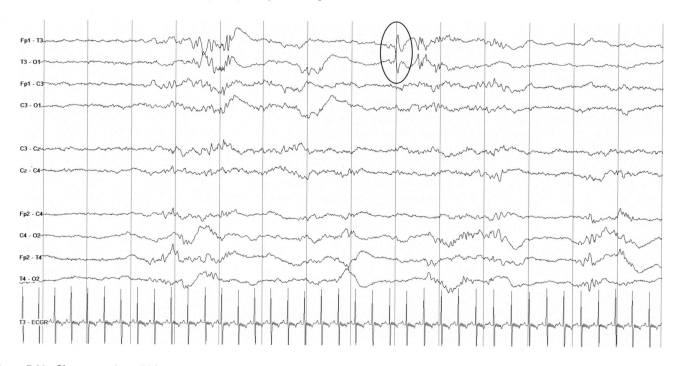

Figure 5.14　Sharp transient. EEG showing left temporal sharp transient. This sharp activity is considered of unknown significance and should not be considered abnormal unless it is very frequent or with persistent focal localization.

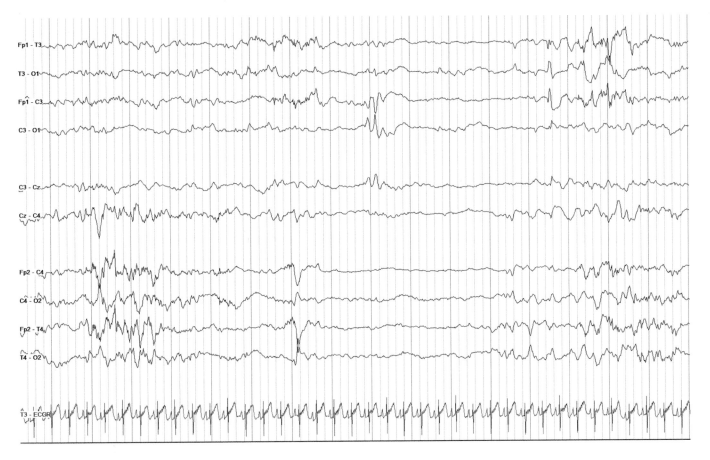

Figure 5.15 Pathological sharp transients. EEG showing multifocal sharp waves.

Table 5.6   Difference between sharp waves seen in the neonatal period

Characteristic	Frontal sharp waves (encoche frontales)	Physiologic sharp transients	Central positive sharp transients
Significance	Normal	Unknown[a]	Associated with white matter injury
Amplitude	High amplitude (50–150 μV)	<75 μV	50–250 μV
Duration	200 ms	<100 ms	>150 ms
Most frequent localization	Frontal, bilateral and synchronous	Any region	Central regions
Sleep/Awake cycle	Sleep	Sleep	Sleep and wakefulness
Frequency		1–2/minute[a]	Several per hour
Occurrence	34–44 weeks CA, usually isolated, but may happen in runs	Isolated	Single or in runs
Morphology	Diphasic	Mono or diphasic	Polyphasic
Polarity	Surface negative followed by surface positive	Surface negative	Surface positive

Note: CA: conceptional age.
[a] If they occur in runs or in excessive frequency, they should be considered pathologic.

transients are not well defined, but if they are surface positive, occur in runs, have specific focal localization, or are excessively frequent, they should be classified as pathological (Tsuchida *et al.*, 2013) **Table 5.6**.

Pathological sharp transients (either positive or negative) are associated with underlying brain dysfunction; however, they do not typically correlate with an increased chance of seizures arising from the underlying cortex, therefore they are not described as epileptiform.

Sharp frontal transients (encoche frontales) should be considered as abnormal if they appear after 6 weeks post term, or occur in long runs, are very frequent, have atypical morphology, persistent unilateral predominance or are seen during wakefulness.

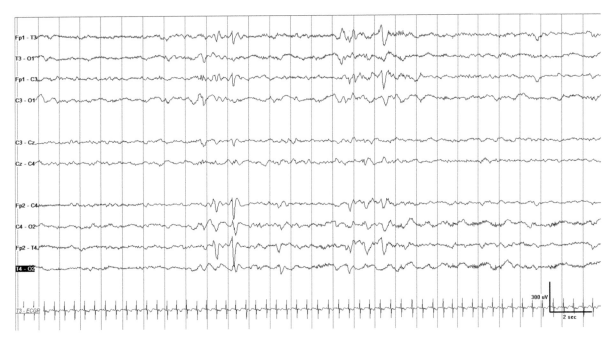

Figure 5.16   Pathological sharp transients. EEG of a term baby showing frequent sharp waves over the frontal regions. Also note abnormal discontinuity for age.

SEIZURES

Synaptogenesis and myelination are incomplete in the immature brain, which precludes the occurrence of generalized seizures except in rare, catastrophic neonatal epileptic encephalopathies. Neonatal seizures are almost always focal and often characterized by paroxysmal events that can be clinically subtle; therefore, their clinical diagnosis is difficult, and video-EEG is the gold standard.

Neonatal seizures can present the same electrographic pattern presented by older patients with focal seizures, characterized by rhythmic sharp waves that gradually increase in

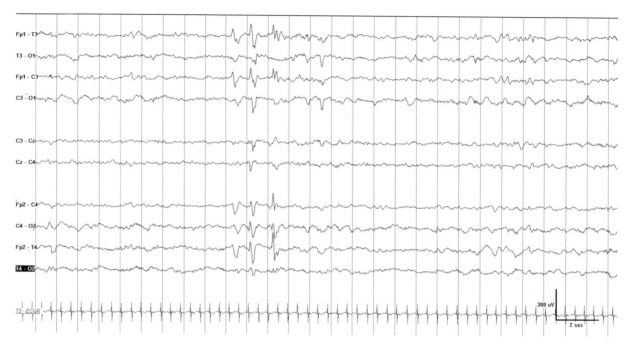

Figure 5.17   Pathological sharp transients. EEG of a term baby showing frequent sharp waves over the frontal regions.

amplitude and decrease in frequency (**Figures 5.18** and **5.19**). However, sometimes neonatal seizures can begin abruptly and have a constant wave morphology throughout the whole event (Mizrahi & Hrachovy, 2016). In addition, the lack of myelination and synaptogenesis restricts the discharge to the same area, without spreading to adjacent brain regions. These features are important to be considered because the absence of "evolution" and a "field" can be interpreted as electrode artifacts by inexperienced neurophysiologists.

Electrographic seizures are common in the neonatal period, and they are characterized by "sudden, repetitive, evolving stereotyped waveforms with a definite beginning, middle, and end with a minimum duration of 10 seconds" (Clancy *et al.*, 1988).

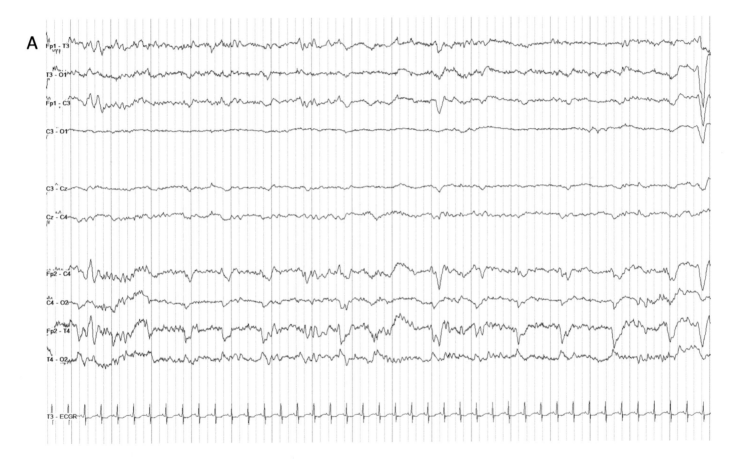

Figure 5.18   (A–C) Neonatal seizure. (A) EEG showing a focal seizure in the right hemisphere characterized by rhythmic sharply contoured waves that, as the seizure evolves (B and C), become more rhythmic and with a sharper morphology. *(Continued)*

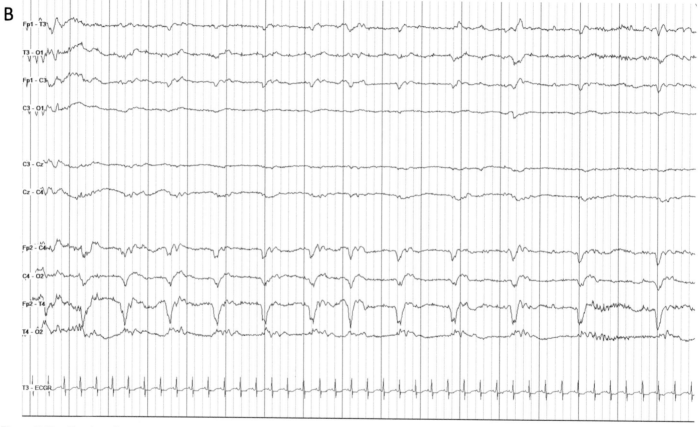

Figure 5.18   *(Continued)*

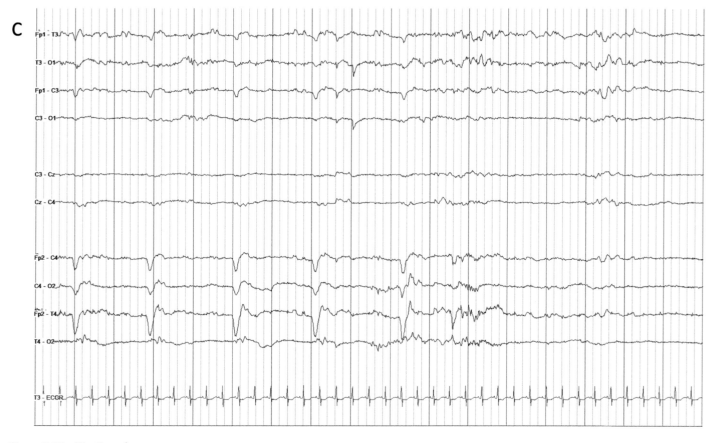

Figure 5.18 *(Continued)*

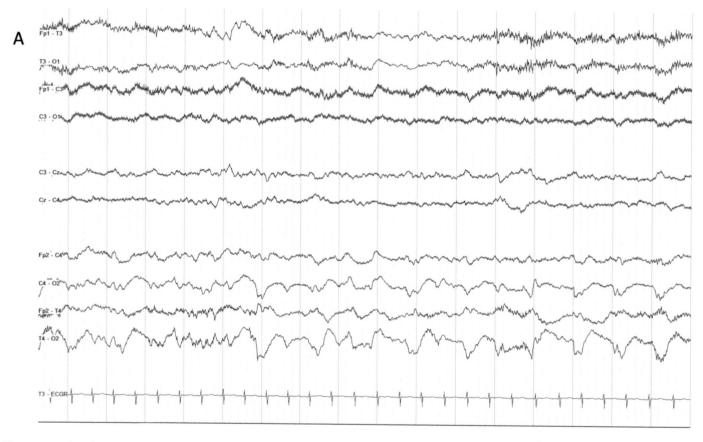

Figure 5.19   (A–C) Neonatal seizure. (A) EEG showing a focal seizure in the right hemisphere characterized by rhythmic sharply contoured waves that, as the seizure evolves (B and C), become more rhythmic and with a sharper morphology.

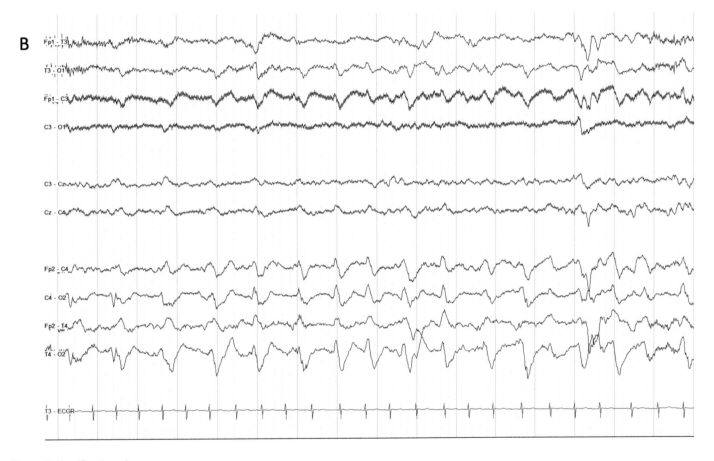

Figure 5.19 *(Continued)*

C

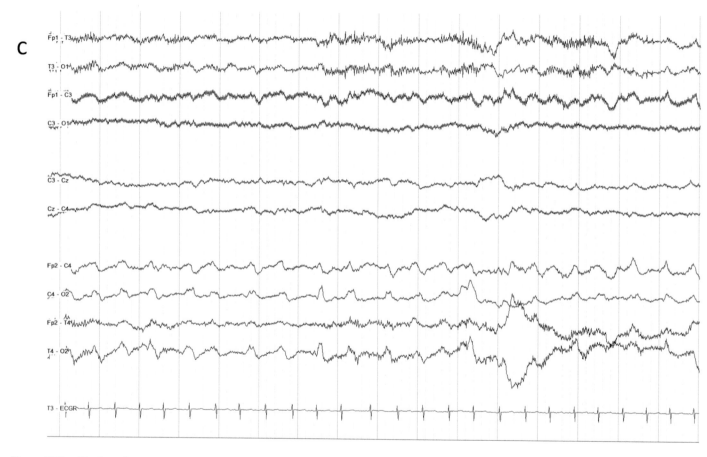

Figure 5.19   *(Continued)*

The 10 seconds necessary to characterize an electrographic seizure is arbitrary and some authors argue that several clinical seizures are shorter than 10 seconds at any age. In addition, neonatal seizures have unique characteristics and do not fit the classical characteristics of seizures presented by older children and adults. But most neurophysiologists agree that if a subclinical rhythmic discharge lasts 10 seconds (or longer) it should be classified as an electrographic seizure. Rhythmic discharges with a shorter duration are classified as brief rhythmic discharges (BRDs; also called brief interictal/ictal rhythmic discharges: BIRDs).

Brief rhythmic discharges (BRDs) are runs of sharply contoured rhythmic activity, with or without evolution, lasting less than 10 seconds (**Figures 5.20** and **5.21**). It is associated

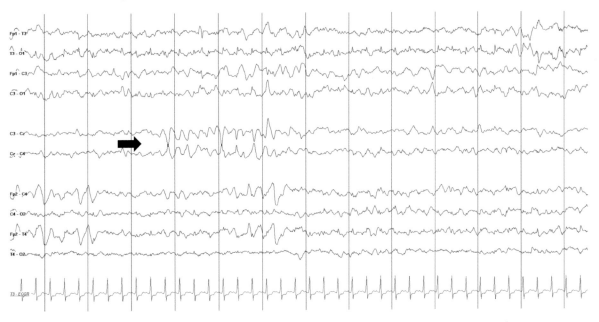

Figure 5.20   Brief rhythmic discharge (BRD). EEG of a 3-day-old term baby showing a run of sharply contoured rhythmic activity over the central region lasting two seconds.

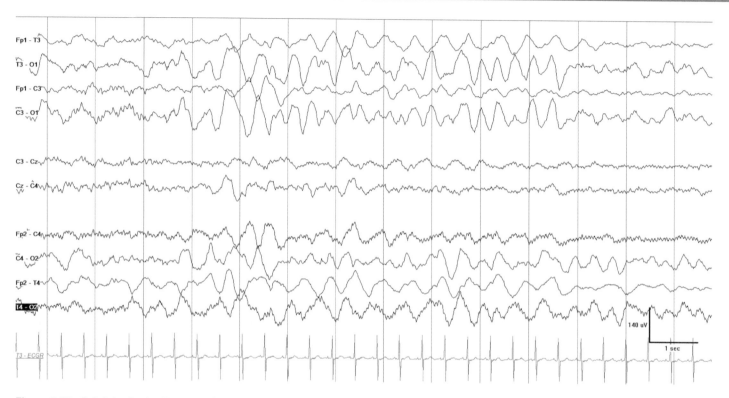

Figure 5.21   Brief rhythmic discharge (BRD). EEG during coma showing an 8 second run of high amplitude sharply contoured delta over the left hemisphere with a field over the homologous contralateral region.

with electrographic seizures with the same morphology in the same or subsequent EEG recordings (Oliveira *et al.*, 2000; Yoo *et al.*, 2014). BRDs may be considered part of the ictal-interictal continuum; and when there is clear evolution it might represent a brief seizure (Pressler *et al.*, 2021).

MONITORIZATION OF ENCEPHALOPATHY SEVERITY

Serial EEG monitorization can be useful in the evaluation of the degree of neonatal encephalopathy. Unfavorable EEG findings associated with poor prognosis are burst-suppression, low voltage, persistent asymmetry, and asynchrony. One of the most reliable favorable signs is the return of sleep states cycling (Holmes & Lombroso, 1993).

Self-Limited Neonatal Epilepsy (SeLNE)

- Age: Usually between 2 and 7 days of life.
- Seizure type: Focal tonic or focal clonic, usually affecting the head, face, or limbs. Lateralization can change.
- Former names: Benign neonatal seizures or convulsions.
- EEG findings: Normal background (may have mild background slowing), interictal sharp waves in the central, centrotemporal, or frontotemporal areas. Ictal: usually focal attenuation of the EEG lasting several seconds, followed by repetitive rhythmic spikes (Cornet *et al.*, 2021; Zuberi *et al.*, 2022).

Self-limited familial neonatal-infantile epilepsy (SeLFNIE)

- Age: Usually between 2 days of life and 7 months.
- Seizure type: Focal tonic or focal clonic, usually in head, face, or limbs. Lateralization can change. May occur in clusters.
- Former names: Benign familial neonatal seizures or convulsions.
- EEG findings: Normal background (may have mild background slowing), interictal spikes, mostly at posterior regions (Herlenius *et al.*, 2007).

Early-infantile developmental and epileptic encephalopathy (EIDEE)

- Onset: Usually neonatal period, up to 3 months old.
- Seizure type: Myoclonic, focal tonic, focal clonic, epileptic spasms.
- Former names: This syndrome includes patients with Ohtahara syndrome and early myoclonic encephalopathy (Zuberi *et al.*, 2022). Although these two syndromes used to be classified separately as two different disorders based on their electroclinical features, there are considerable overlap and even similar etiologies.
- EEG: Low-voltage background, burst-suppression, multifocal spikes/sharp waves (**Figure 5.22**).

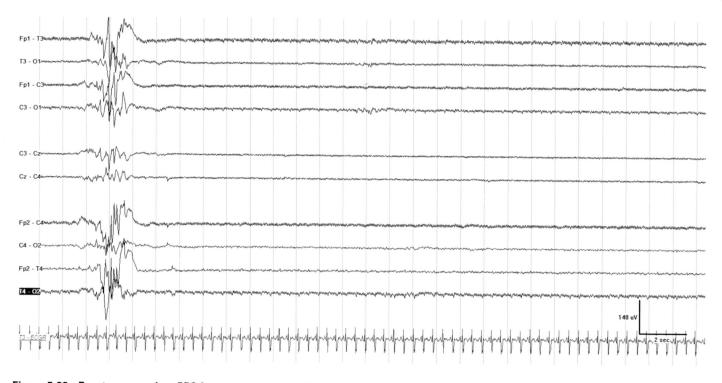

Figure 5.22   Burst-suppression. EEG from a term neonate with early-infantile developmental and epileptic encephalopathy showing high-amplitude generalized polyspikes followed by diffuse voltage suppression for several seconds.

REFERENCES

Clancy RR, Legido A, Lewis D. Occult Neonatal Seizures. Epilepsia 1988;29:256–61.

Cornet MC, Morabito V, Lederer D, et al. Neonatal Presentation of Genetic Epilepsies: Early Differentiation from Acute Provoked Seizures. Epilepsia 2021;62:1907–20.

Herlenius E, Heron SE, Grinton BE, et al. SCN2A Mutations and Benign Familial Neonatal-Infantile Seizures: The Phenotypic Spectrum. Epilepsia 2007;48:1138–42.

Holmes G, Lombroso C. Prognostic Value of Background Patterns in the Neonatal EEG. J Clin Neirophysiol 1993;10:323–52.

Mizrahi EM, Hrachovy RA. Atlas of Neonatal Electroencephalography. 4th Ed. New York: Demos Medical; 2016.

Oliveira AJ, Nunes ML, Haertel LM, Reis FM, da Costa JC. Duration of Rhythmic EEG Patterns in Neonates: New Evidence for Clinical and Prognostic Significance of Brief Rhythmic Discharges. Clin Neurophysiol 2000;111:1646–53.

Pressler RM, Cilio MR, Mizrahi EM, et al. The ILAE Classification of Seizures and the Epilepsies: Modification for Seizures in the Neonate.

Position Paper by the ILAE Task Force on Neonatal Seizures. Epilepsia 2021;62:615–28.

Shellhaas RA, Chang T, Tsuchida T, et al. The American Clinical Neurophysiology Society's Guideline on Continuous Electroencephalography Monitoring in Neonates. J Clin Neurophysiol 2011;28:611–17.

Tsuchida TN, Wusthoff CJ, Shellhaas RA, et al. American Clinical Neurophysiology Society Standardized EEG Terminology and Categorization for the Description of Continuous EEG Monitoring in Neonates: Report of the American Clinical Neurophysiology Society Critical Care Monitoring Committee. J Clin Neurophysiol 2013;30:161–73.

Yoo JY, Rampal N, Petroff OA, Hirsch LJ, Gaspard N. Brief Potentially Ictal Rhythmic Discharges in Critically Ill Adults. JAMA Neurol 2014;71:454–62.

Zuberi SM, Wirrell E, Yozawitz E, et al. ILAE Classification and Definition of Epilepsy Syndromes with Onset in Neonates and Infants: Position Statement by the ILAE Task Force on Nosology and Definitions. Epilepsia 2022;63:1349–97.

CHAPTER 6

Normal wakefulness

Aliya Frederick, MD, PhD

Maria Augusta Montenegro, MD, PhD

After the newborn period, the EEG during wakefulness should be continuous, characterized by diffuse delta and theta waves. After a few months, the anterior-posterior gradient starts to be more evident. As the child gets older, the background shifts toward faster frequencies, with more theta, alpha, and beta present, depending upon the age of the child.

As in adults, the awake background in children is characterized by an anterior-posterior gradient, comprised of an admixture of rhythms with posteriorly predominant alpha (or slower frequencies in young children) and anteriorly predominant beta. The posterior dominant rhythm varies according to the patient's age, and as the brain matures, the posterior dominant rhythm gets faster. Most children will have a posterior dominant rhythm of 8 Hz at 3 years old (**Figures 6.1–6.14**), however, sometimes, a slower frequency may be seen without it

being considered abnormal. At 8 years old, the child must have a posterior dominant rhythm of at least 8 Hz (Gibbs & Knott, 1949; **Table 6.1**).

Table 6.1 Posterior dominant rhythm according to each age

Age	Common PDR frequency	Minimally required PDR
1 year-old	6	5
2 years-old	7	5
3 years-old	8	6
5 years-old	9	7
8 years-old	9	8
10 years-old	10	8

Note: PDR: posterior dominant rhythm.

DOI: 10.1201/b23339-6

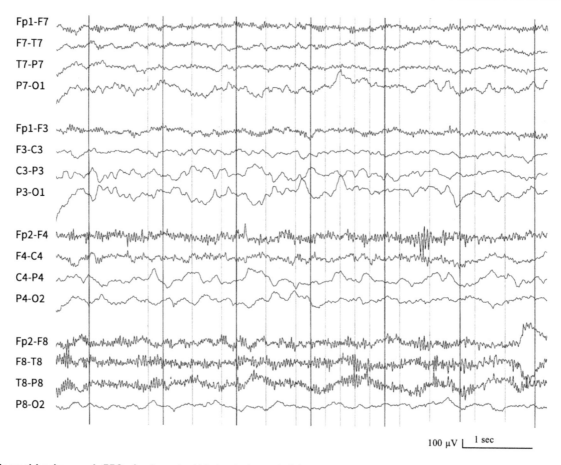

Figure 6.1   Normal background. EEG of a 6-week-old baby during wakefulness showing continuous admixture of theta and delta range waves. Progressively, the theta range waves substitute the delta waves and the posterior dominant rhythm is more evident.

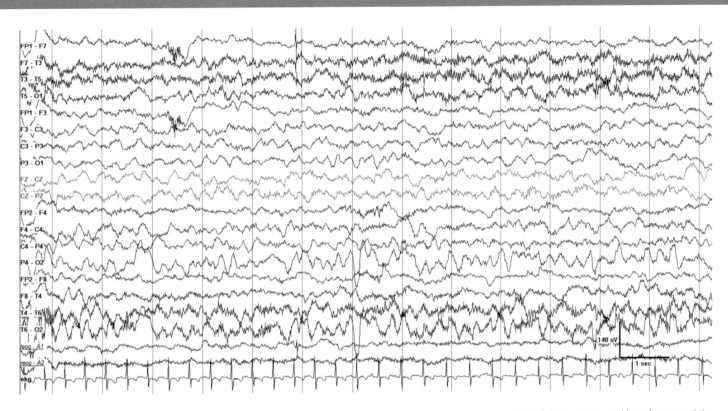

Figure 6.2   Normal background. EEG of a 3-month-old baby during wakefulness showing higher proportion of theta waves and less frequent delta range waves.

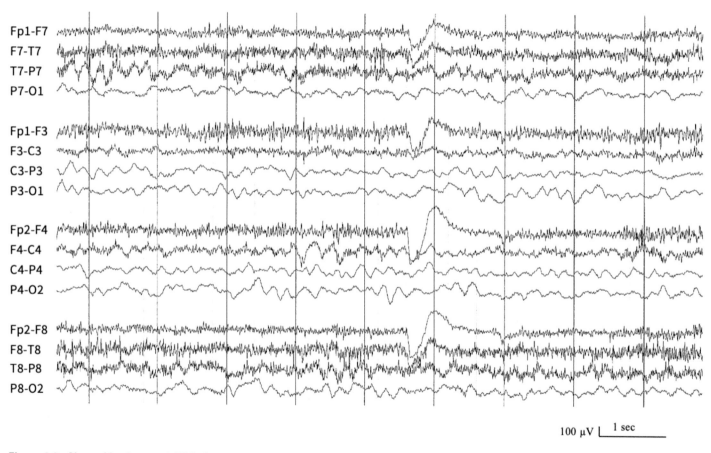

100 µV | 1 sec

Figure 6.3   Normal background. EEG of a 4-month-old baby during wakefulness showing continuous theta range frequencies and a posterior dominant rhythm of 4 to 5 Hz.

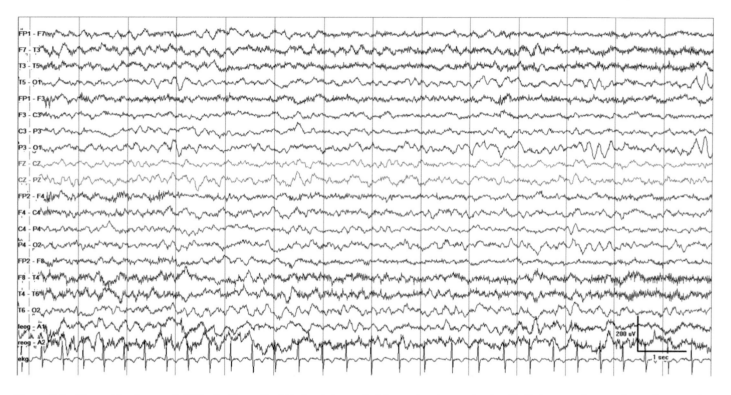

Figure 6.4   Normal background. EEG of a 7-month-old baby during wakefulness showing predominantly theta range frequencies and a posterior dominant rhythm of 4 to 5 Hz.

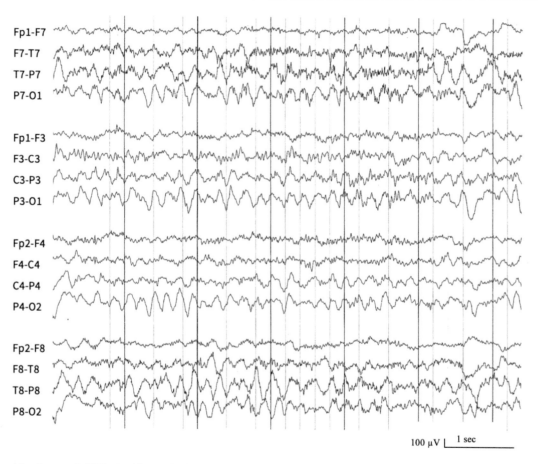

Figure 6.5   Normal background. EEG of a 10-month-old baby during wakefulness showing predominantly theta range frequencies and a posterior dominant rhythm of 6 Hz.

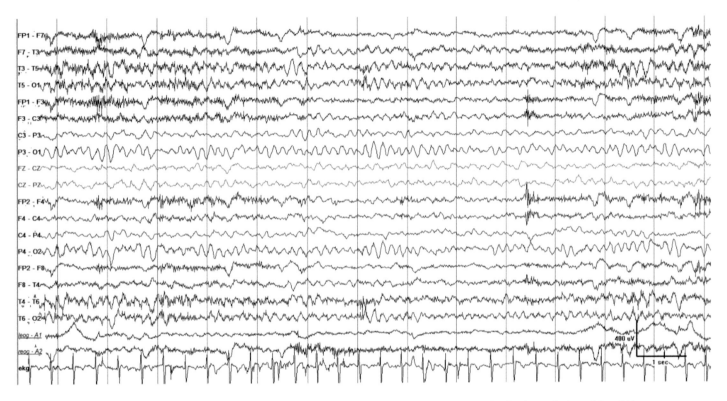

Figure 6.6   Normal background. EEG of a 15-month-old baby during wakefulness showing a posterior dominant rhythm of 6 to 7 Hz.

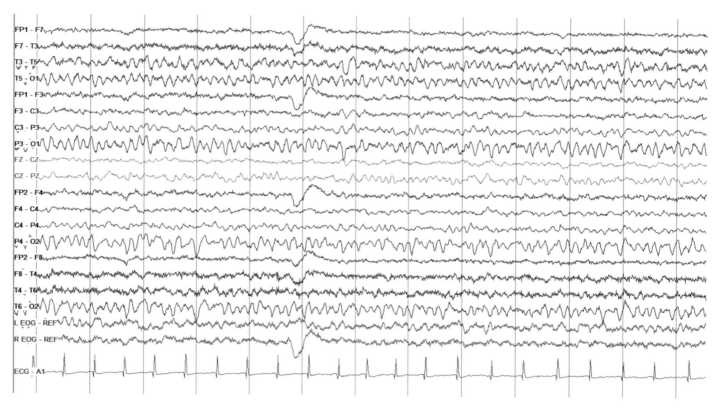

Figure 6.7   Normal background. EEG of a 2-year-old girl during wakefulness showing a posterior dominant rhythm of 7 Hz.

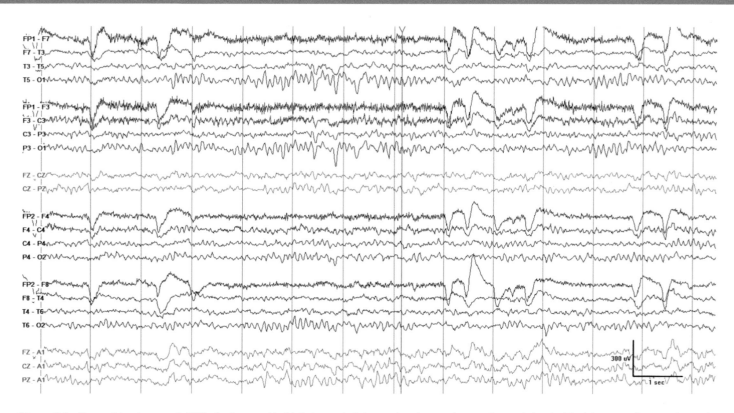

Figure 6.8   Normal background. EEG of a 3-year-old girl during wakefulness showing continuous theta admixed with alpha range frequencies and a posterior dominant rhythm of 9 Hz.

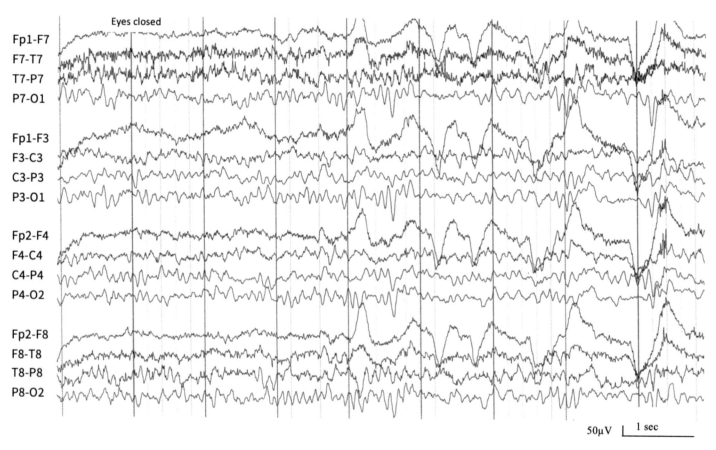

Figure 6.9   Normal background. EEG of a 6-year-old boy during wakefulness showing continuous theta frequencies admixed with alpha range potentials and a posterior dominant rhythm of 9 Hz.

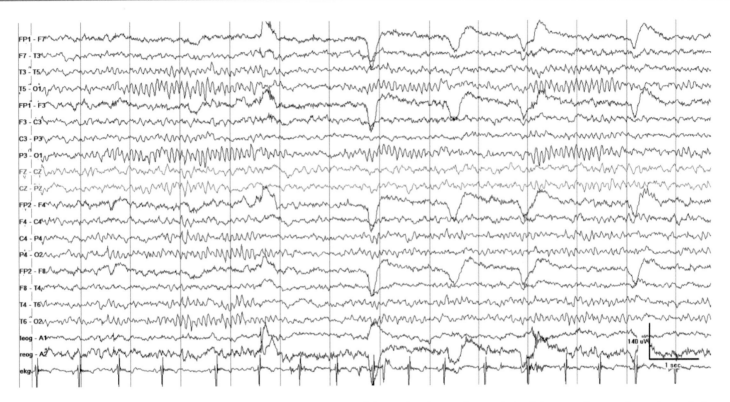

Figure 6.10   Normal background. EEG of a 9-year-old girl during wakefulness showing continuous theta-alpha range frequencies and a posterior dominant rhythm of 10 Hz. There is good posterior dominant rhythm reactivity to eye-opening.

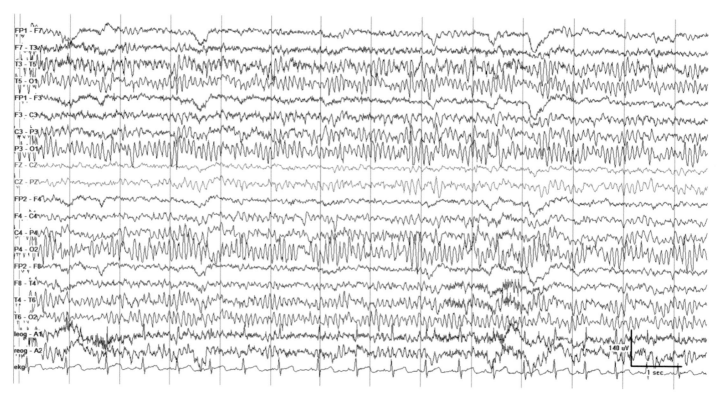

Figure 6.11   Normal background. EEG of a 12-year-old boy during wakefulness showing a posterior dominant rhythm of 10 Hz. At this age, the posterior dominant rhythm has a high amplitude and sharp appearance.

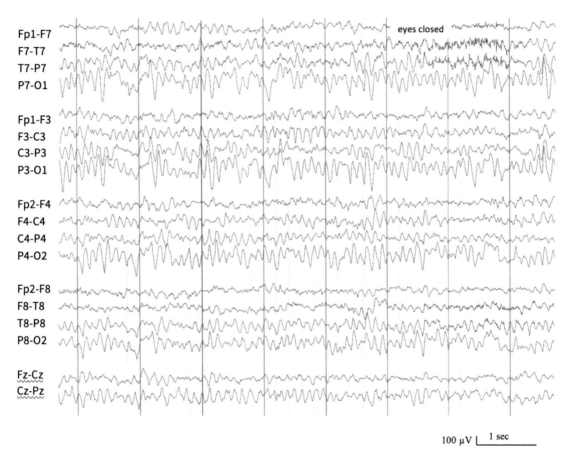

Figure 6.12   Normal background. EEG of a 14-year-old boy during wakefulness showing a posterior dominant rhythm of 9–10 Hz. At this age, the posterior dominant rhythm has a high amplitude and sharp appearance.

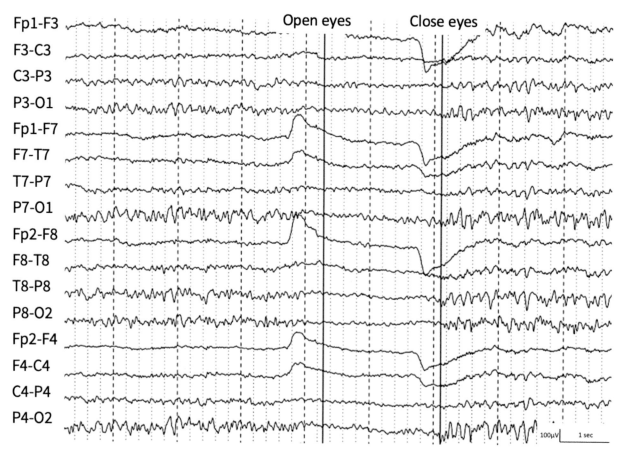

Figure 6.13   Reactivity of the posterior dominant rhythm to eye-opening and closure. EEG showing that the posterior dominant rhythm disappears after eye-opening and comes back after eye closure. Note that the right hemisphere (non-dominant hemisphere) has a slightly higher amplitude. Also note the anterior-posterior gradient with posteriorly predominant alpha and anteriorly predominant beta.

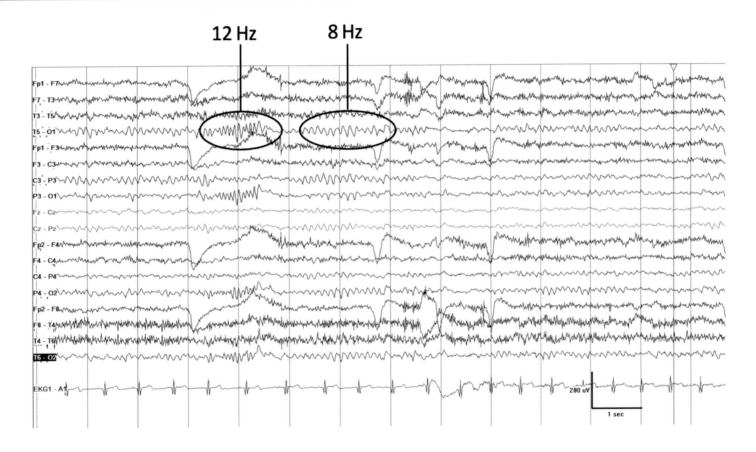

Figure 6.14 Alpha squeak. The posterior dominant rhythm is faster immediately after eye closure (alpha squeak); therefore, the baseline posterior dominant rhythm frequency should not be assessed immediately after eye closure.

The posterior dominant rhythm should be reactive to eye-opening and closure starting at 3 to 4 months of age (Riviello *et al.*, 2011). Because it is faster for 0.5 to 1 second immediately after eye closure (alpha squeak), the baseline frequency of the patient should not be assessed immediately after eye closure (**Figures 6.13** and **6.14**).

The amplitude of the posterior dominant rhythm varies from individual to individual, and even in the same patient (Chang *et al.*, 2011). In adults, the posterior dominant rhythm has an amplitude between 40 and 50μV, and higher amplitudes are frequently seen in younger patients. Mild posterior dominant rhythm asymmetry is considered normal, with higher amplitudes typically seen in the non-dominant hemisphere. Amplitude asymmetry greater than 50% should be carefully evaluated, and if it is present in at least two montages (one referential and one bipolar), it might represent an abnormality (Markand, 1990). It is important to note that symmetry applies only to the amplitude and frequency of the waves; and synchrony refers to the presence of these descriptors occurring simultaneously between the two hemispheres (Hirsch *et al.*, 2022).

Posterior slow waves of youth are square-shaped delta waves seen over the posterior regions in the same region of the posterior dominant rhythm. This is a normal finding that can occur unilaterally or bilaterally and they are usually seen from the second half of the first decade until adolescence (**Figures 6.15** and **6.16**). Slow waves of youth are seen with eyes closed and are blocked by eye-opening.

The *mu* rhythm is named after the Greek letter (Mμ) because it is a rhythm strongly related to the motor cortex (**Figures 6.17**–**6.19**). It is recorded in the central regions, does not react to eye-opening or closure, and is suppressed by movement, tactile stimuli, or if the patient thinks about moving the contralateral limb. In adults, it is characterized by sharply contoured waves around 8–12 Hz and is more prominent in the C3 and C4 electrodes. It has a slower frequency in children, ranging from 5 to 7 Hz in the infant with a progressive increase until adolescence (Berchicci *et al.*, 2011; Smith, 1941). The *mu* rhythm is not always seen on routine EEG, and its absence is not considered an abnormality. However, if the *mu* rhythm is consistently unilateral it can be associated with an ipsilateral cortical lesion (Yamak *et al.*, 2017).

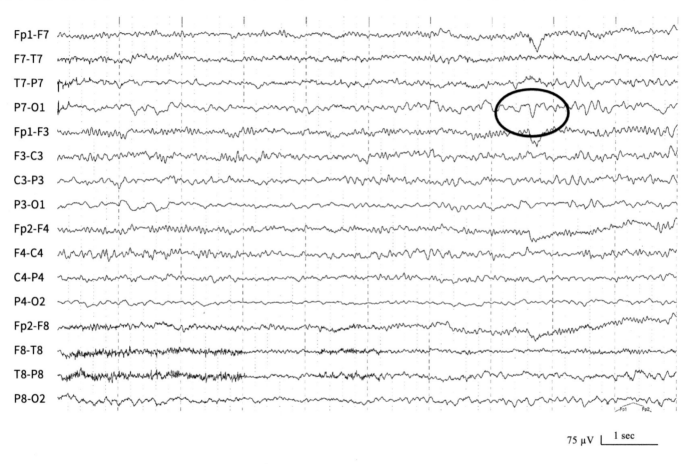

Figure 6.15 Posterior slow waves of youth. Awake EEG showing slow waves in the posterior regions. These potentials occur during wakefulness, usually have a "squared" morphology and can last for several seconds in duration.

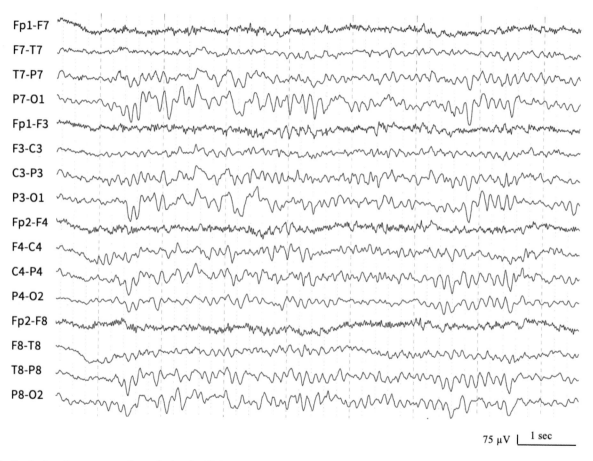

75 µV | 1 sec

Figure 6.16 Posterior slow waves of youth. Awake EEG showing slow waves in the posterior regions. These potentials occur during wakefulness, usually have a "squared" morphology, and can last for several seconds in duration.

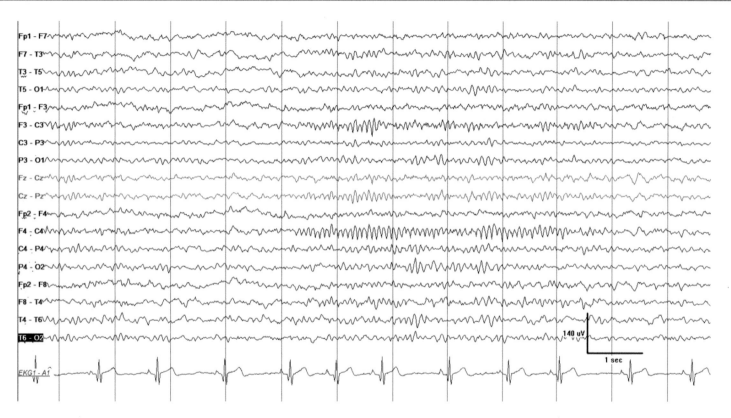

Figure 6.17   *Mu* rhythm. Awake EEG showing sharply contoured waves in the alpha frequency, more prominent in the central region.

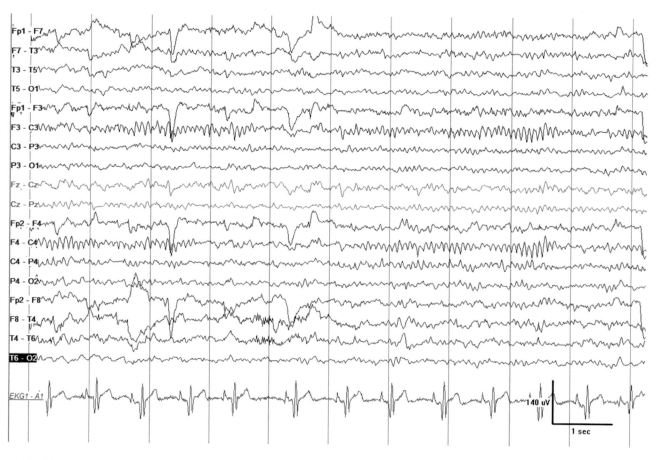

Figure 6.18   *Mu* rhythm. Awake EEG showing sharply contoured alpha frequencies in the central regions.

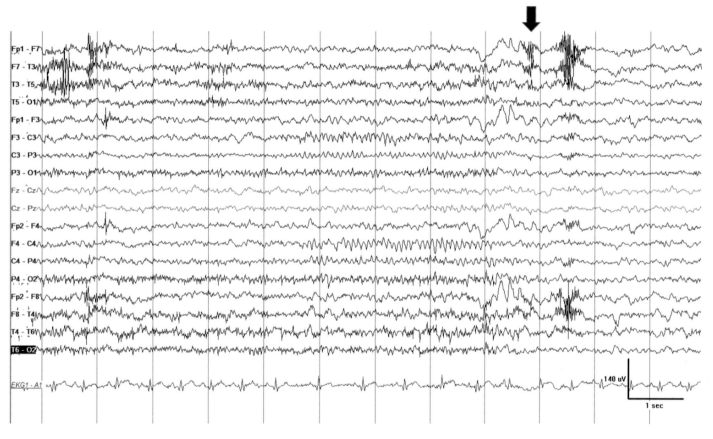

Figure 6.19 *Mu* **rhythm.** Awake EEG showing sharply contoured alpha frequencies in the central regions. Note that when the patient moves (arrow indicating muscle artifact), the *mu* rhythm disappears.

REFERENCES

Berchicci M, Zhang T, Romero L, Peters A, Annett R, Teuscher U, Bertollo M, Okada Y, Stephen J, Comani S. Development of *mu rhythm* in Infants and Preschool Children. Dev Neurosci 2011;33:130–43.

Chang BS, Schomer DL, Niedermeyer E. Normal EEG and Sleep: Adults and Elderly. In: Schomer, DL, da Silva, FHL (Eds). Niedermeyer's Electroencephalography: Basic Principles, Clinical Applications, and Related Fields, 6th Ed. Philadelphia: Lippincott Williams & Wilkins; 2011. p. 358–430.

Gibbs FA, Knott JR. Growth of the Electrical Activity of the Cortex. Electroencephalogr Clin Neurophysiol 1949;1:223–29.

Hirsch E, French J, Scheffer IE, et al. ILAE Definition of the Idiopathic Generalized Epilepsy Syndromes: Position Statement by the ILAE Task Force on Nosology and Definitions. Epilepsia 2022;63:1475–99.

Markand OM. Alpha Rhythms. J Clin Neurophysiol 1990;7:163–89.

Riviello JJ Jr, Nordli DR Jr, Niedermeyer E. Normal EEG and Sleep: Infants and Adolescents. In: Schomer, DL, da Silva, FHL (Eds). Niedermeyer's Electroencephalography: Basic Principles, Clinical Applications, and Related Fields, 6th Ed. Philadelphia: Lippincott Williams & Wilkins; 2011. p. 321–57.

Smith JR. The Frequency Growth of the Human Alpha Rhythms during Normal Infancy and Childhood. J Physiol 1941;11:177–98.

Yamak WR, Beydoun AA, Dirani MM, Toufaili HA, El Hajj TI, Nasreddine WM. Unilateral *mu rhythm* and Associated Cortical Lesions on Brain MRI. J Clin Neurophysiol 2017;34:144–50.

Chapter 7

Normal sleep

Maria Augusta Montenegro, MD, PhD

Important maturational milestones should be considered when reading pediatric sleep EEG. Neonatal sleep patterns (beta-delta complexes, *tracé alternant*, etc.) disappear after 46–48 weeks of conceptional age (Riviello *et al.*, 2011), and after this age, sleep should be an admixture of continuous theta and delta waves. Spindles, vertex waves, and K complex appear during the first months of life, and both the number of hours of sleep per day and the amount of REM sleep will decrease during the first year of life (**Figure 7.1**).

Like in adults, drowsiness is characterized by posterior dominant rhythm waxing and waning attenuation followed by the appearance of diffuse medium to high-amplitude theta range waves (**Figures 7.2–7.5**). During the first year of life and throughout the first decade and early teenage years, hypnagogic hypersynchrony can appear in drowsiness. It is characterized by paroxysmal high-amplitude sinusoidal theta waves (**Figures 7.6** and **7.7**). Hypnopompic hypersynchrony (or arousal reaction)

has the same characteristics of hypnagogic hypersynchrony but is seen during arousal (**Figures 7.8** and **7.9**). It is rare in adults.

Sleep spindles appear around 6 weeks of age and should be present in every infant at 2 months of age (**Figures 7.10–7.15**). In the neonatal period, sleep onset is characterized by REM sleep, and there is a gradual evolution to non-REM sleep at sleep onset in the following weeks/months. In the first months of life, the absence of spindles in a routine EEG should be carefully evaluated if the recording has a short duration because it may include only REM sleep (Riviello *et al.*, 2011). Around 3 months of age, spindles have a very long duration, up to several seconds. As the baby grows, spindles become shorter and should be synchronous at 24 months of age (due to the maturation of the thalamocortical commissural pathways; Hughes, 1994; **Table 7.1**).

Although extreme spindles have a morphology similar to sleep spindles, they represent different EEG elements. When compared to sleep spindles, extreme spindles are recorded mostly in children, have a

DOI: 10.1201/b23339-7

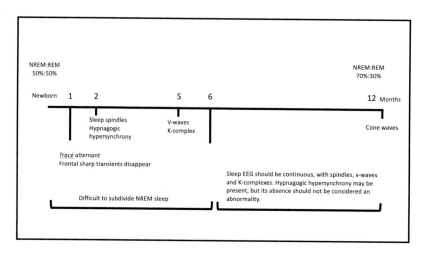

Figure 7.1   Sleep maturation in the first year of life.

Table 7.1   Sleep spindles evolution from infancy to adulthood

Characteristics	Children	Adolescent/adult
Localization	More anterior (frontal)	Central
Length	Very long in the first months of life	Only a few seconds
Frequency	14 Hz	11–12 Hz
Morphology	Arciform, comb-shaped	Sinusoidal
Amplitude	High amplitude	Amplitude decreases with age
Synchrony	Asynchronous (up to 24 months old)	Synchronous

higher amplitude, very long duration (several seconds), predominate in the frontocentral regions, and can also be recorded during wakefulness (**Figure 7.16**). Although controversial, most authors agree that extreme spindles do not represent a normal feature and can be associated with developmental delay, cognitive impairment, and other neurological conditions. In addition, they do not correlate with an increased risk of epilepsy (Gibbs & Gibbs, 1962).

Vertex waves, or v-waves, appear in drowsiness and should be seen in all infants at 5 months of age. In childhood, they may be very sharp and appear in runs (**Figures 7.17** and **7.18**). It may also be anteriorly displaced, over the frontocentral regions (some authors use the term f-wave to describe a frontally predominant vertex wave).

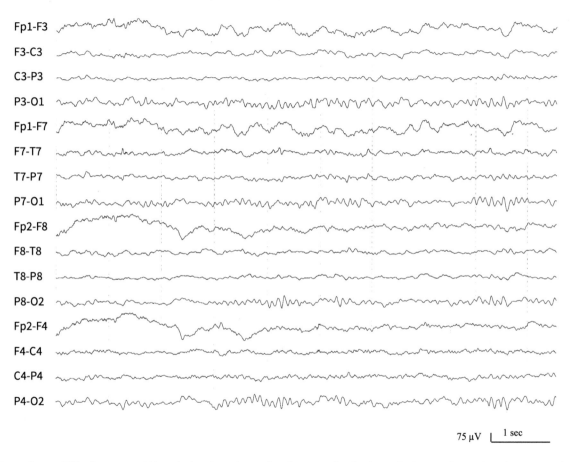

75 µV | 1 sec

Figure 7.2 Drowsiness. EEG of a 4-year-old boy during drowsiness showing posterior dominant rhythm waxing and waning attenuation.

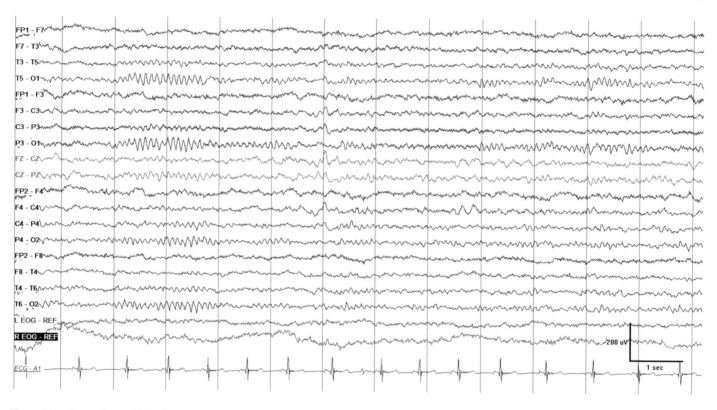

Figure 7.3 **Drowsiness**. EEG of a 9-year-old boy during drowsiness showing posterior dominant rhythm waxing and waning attenuation.

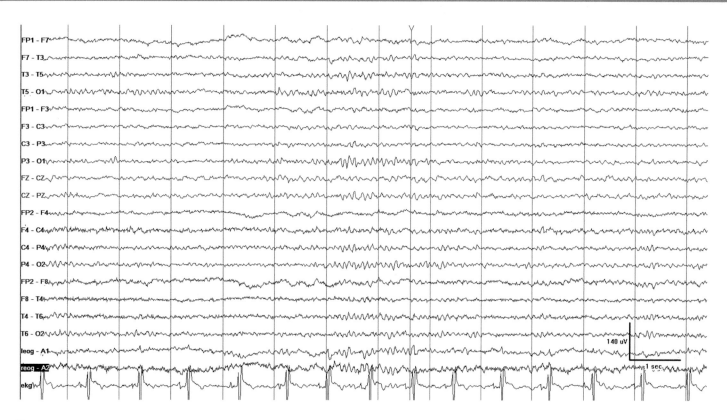

Figure 7.4   Drowsiness. EEG of a 13-year-old girl during drowsiness showing posterior dominant rhythm waxing and waning attenuation.

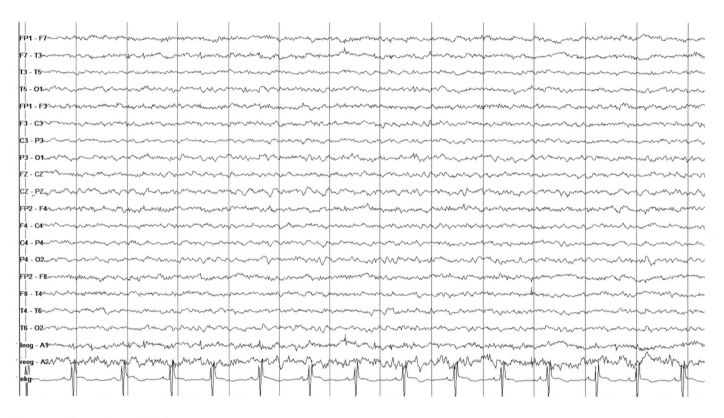

Figure 7.5   Drowsiness. EEG of a 12-year-old boy during drowsiness showing diffuse medium-amplitude theta waves.

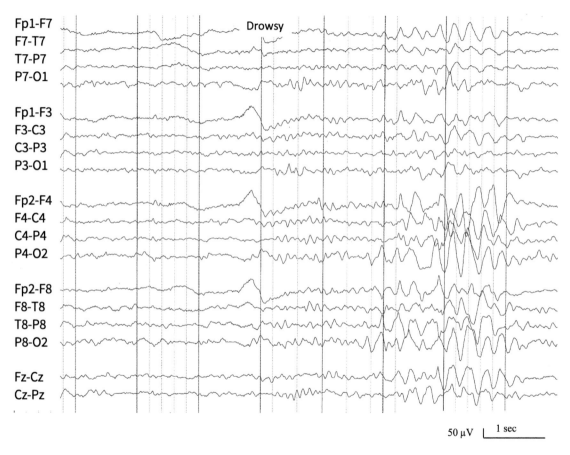

Drowsy

50 μV | 1 sec

Figure 7.6   Hypnagogic hypersynchrony. EEG of a 4-year-old boy showing high-amplitude diffuse sinusoidal theta range waves during drowsiness.

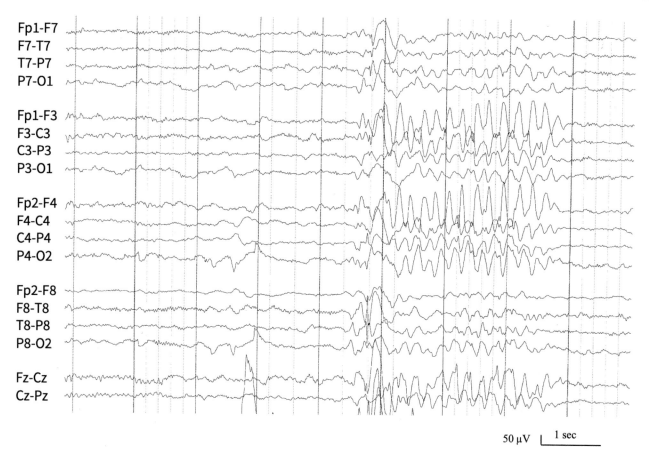

50 μV | 1 sec

Figure 7.7   Hypnagogic hypersynchrony. EEG of a 5-year-old boy showing high-amplitude diffuse sinusoidal theta range waves during drowsiness.

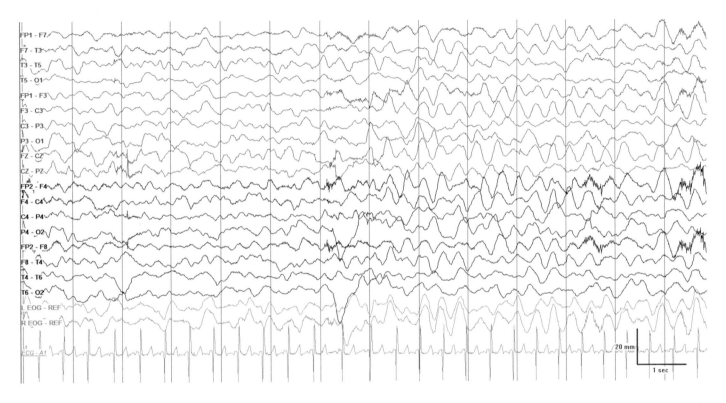

Figure 7.8 Hypnopompic hypersynchrony (arousal reaction). EEG of a 13-month-old boy showing high-amplitude sinusoidal theta waves during arousal.

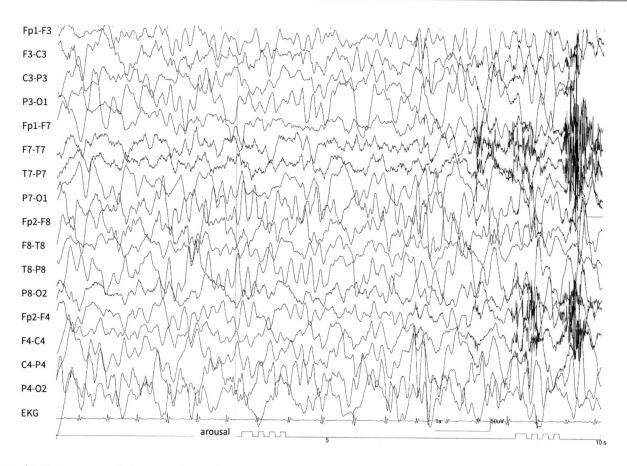

Figure 7.9 (A–C) Hypnopompic hypersynchrony (arousal reaction). EEG of a 4-year-old girl showing rhythmic high-amplitude sinusoidal theta waves during arousal. Note that the event lasts for more than 30 seconds. *(Continued)*

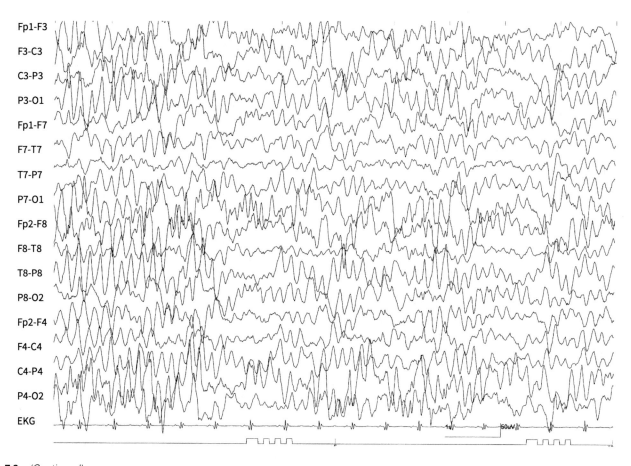

Figure 7.9   *(Continued)*

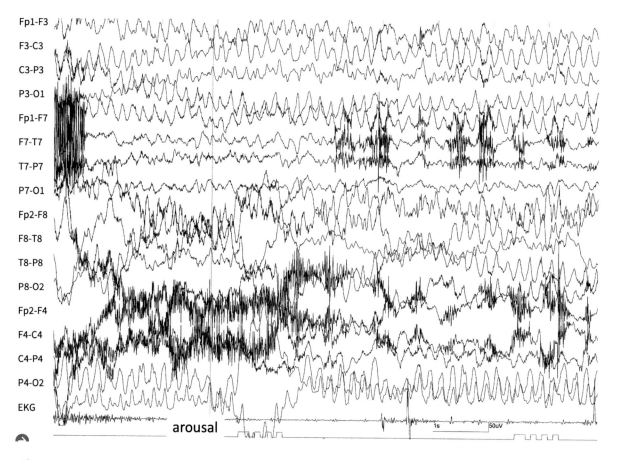

Figure 7.9 *(Continued)*

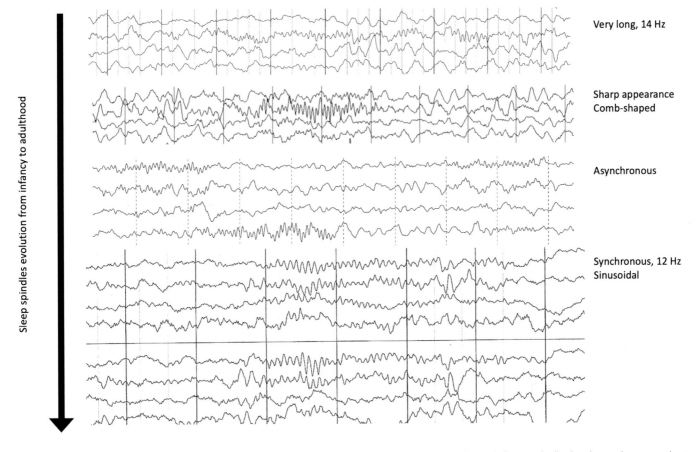

Sleep spindles evolution from infancy to adulthood

Very long, 14 Hz

Sharp appearance
Comb-shaped

Asynchronous

Synchronous, 12 Hz
Sinusoidal

Figure 7.10 Sleep spindles evolution from infancy to adulthood. Note that as the months go by, spindles gradually develop and present shorter duration, slower frequency, become synchronous, and have a more sinusoidal morphology.

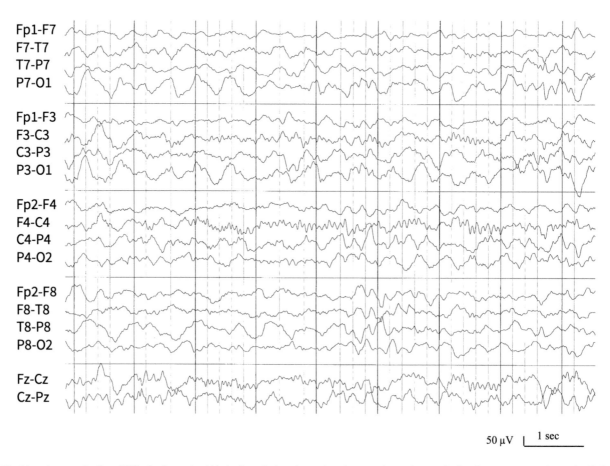

50 μV |⌐ 1 sec

Figure 7.11   Very long spindles. EEG of a 6-week-old baby boy during sleep showing very long sleep spindles (best seen on channel 10). As the baby grows, spindles became of shorter duration and at 24 months of age, they should be synchronous.

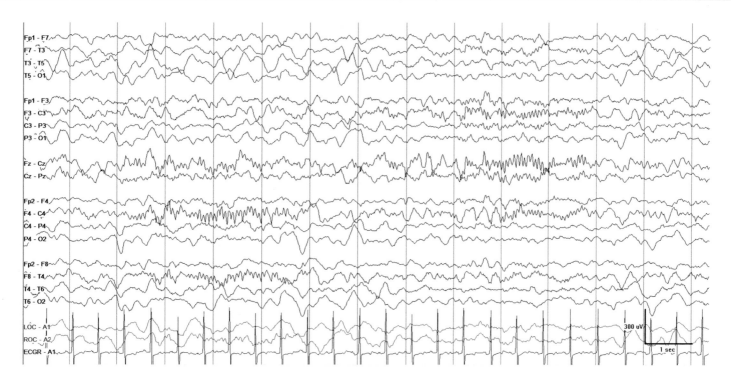

Figure 7.12 Asynchronous spindles. EEG of a 4-month-old baby showing asynchronous sleep spindles, which are normal for this age.

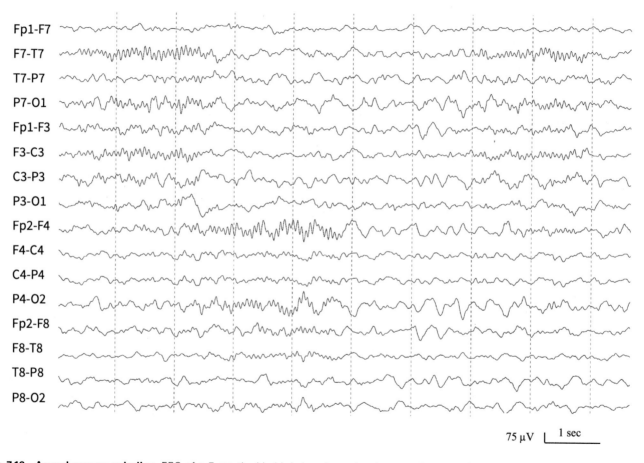

75 μV ⌊ 1 sec

Figure 7.13 Asynchronous spindles. EEG of a 7-month-old girl during sleep showing asynchronous sleep spindles (normal for this age). Sleep spindles should be synchronous at 24 months old.

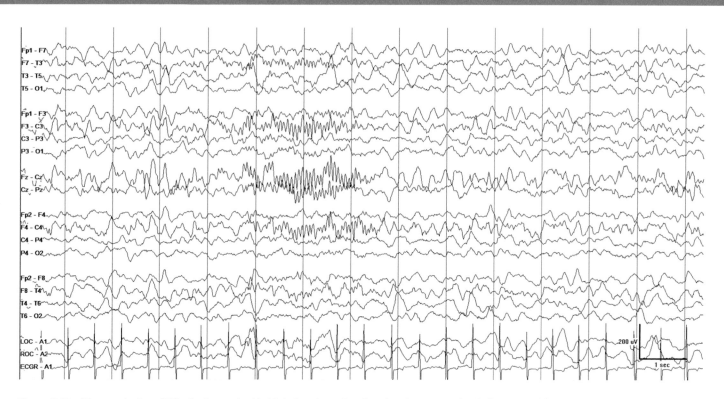

Figure 7.14 Sharp spindles. EEG of a 4-month-old girl during sleep showing sharply contoured spindles, normal for the age.

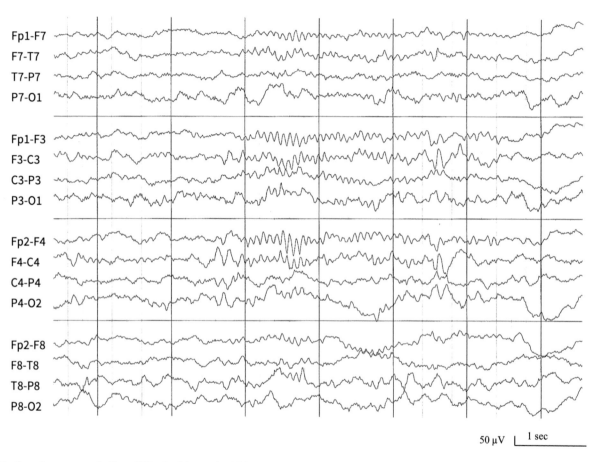

Figure 7.15   Synchronous spindles. EEG of a 24-month-old boy during sleep showing synchronous sleep spindles. Sleep spindles should be synchronous at 24 months old.

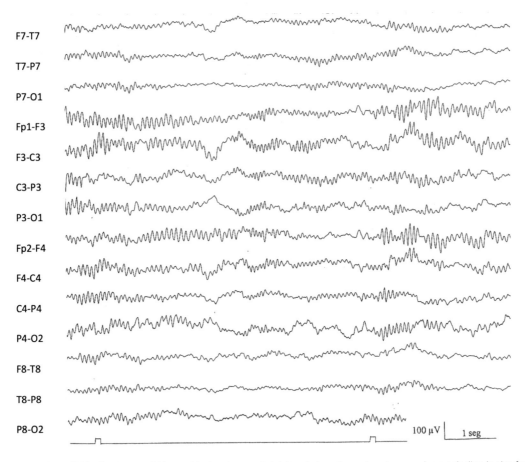

Figure 7.16   Extreme spindles. EEG of a 4-year-old boy with developmental delay during sleep showing very long spindles in the frontocentral regions. (Reprinted from Montenegro *et al.*, 2022, with permission.)

K complexes are a combination of a vertex wave and spindles and also should be seen at 5 months of age. It occurs spontaneously or after a sudden stimulus (**Figures 7.19–7.21**; Amzica & Steriade, 1997).

Although several maturational changes occur during the first years of life, after this period, the characteristics of sleep cycles in a pediatric sleep EEG are not very different from the ones seen in adults. During a full-night sleep, an adult has four to six sleep cycles, each lasting about 90 minutes (the sleep cycles in young children occurs approximately every 60 minutes; Davis *et al.*, 2004). Each sleep cycle has four stages: N1, N2, N3, and REM sleep.

Vertex waves appear in deep drowsiness. The N2 stage (light sleep) shows an admixture of low to moderate theta and delta range waves with vertex waves and sleep spindles in the central region. As the sleep gets deeper (N3 stage), there is a predominance of moderate to high-amplitude delta range waves and a decrease in sleep spindles and vertex waves. REM sleep is characterized by faster frequencies (usually in the alpha range) and horizontal eye-movement artifacts produced by rapid eye movement can be seen over the frontal regions (**Figures 7.22–7.25**). **Table 7.2** and **Figure 7.26** summarize the characteristics of each sleep cycle.

Additional elements that can be seen during the sleep EEG are:

- Occipital slow transients of sleep (cone waves): They are bilateral, high-voltage, cone-shaped occipital delta waves seen during non-REM sleep (**Figures 7.27** and **7.28**). They are seen in young children, especially around 1 to 5 years of age.
- POSTS (positive occipital sharp transients of sleep): They are positive sharp waves seen over the occipital region (**Figure 7.29**).

Table 7.2   Characteristics of each sleep stage

Sleep stage	Physiological characteristics	EEG characteristics
Stage N1 (non-REM)	Drowsiness	Posterior dominant rhythm waxing and waning attenuation. Progressive appearance of diffuse theta range waves. Vertex waves during deep drowsiness. Hypnagogic hypersynchrony.
Stage N2 (non-REM)	Light Sleep Unresponsiveness	Sleep spindles. Vertex waves. K complex. Theta and delta background. POSTS.
Stage N3 (non-REM)	Deep Sleep Unresponsiveness	Spindles and K complex are less frequently seen. Mostly high-amplitude delta background.
REM sleep	Unresponsiveness Muscle atonia Irregular breathing and heart rate REM Dreams	No spindles, vertex waves, or K-complex. Mostly alpha waves.

Abbreviations POSTS: positive occipital sharp transients of sleep; REM: rapid eye movement.

- Mitten: It is a normal variant that occurs during sleep and is characterized by a slow wave with a notch with the same polarity in the frontocentral region. It is a variant of K-complex and v-waves (**Figure 7.30**).

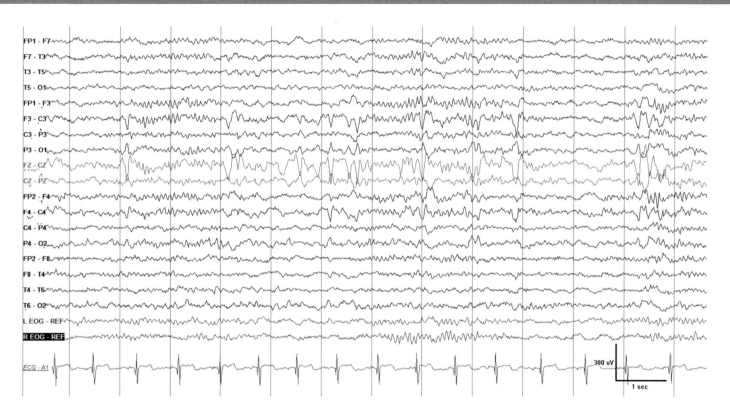

Figure 7.17   Vertex waves. EEG of a 5-year-old girl showing vertex waves in the central region.

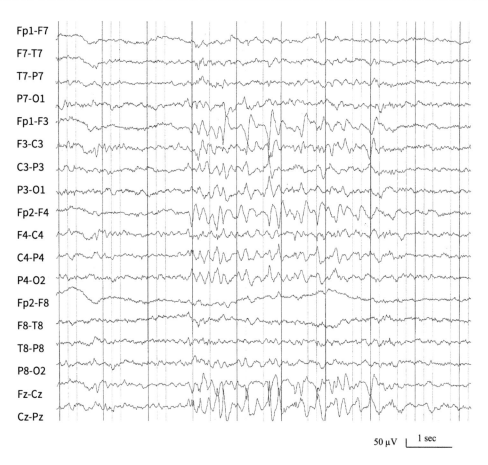

50 μV |__ 1 sec __

Figure 7.18   Vertex waves. EEG of a 9-year-old boy showing a run of sharp vertex waves in the frontocentral region. During childhood, vertex waves can be very sharp and appear in runs. It may also appear a little bit more anteriorly, over the frontocentral regions.

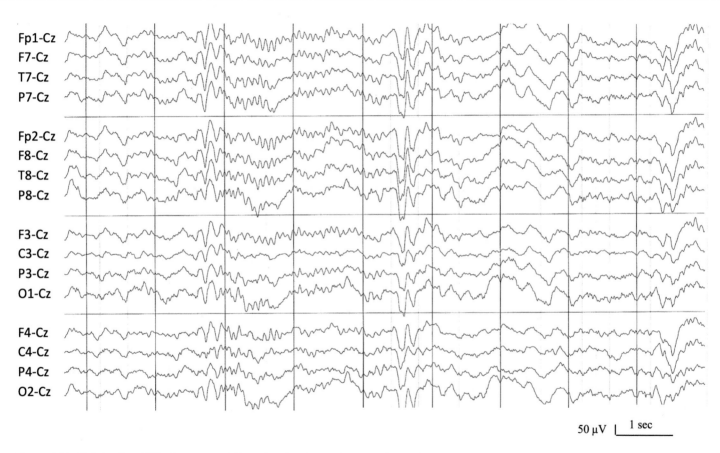

Figure 7.19 K-Complex. EEG of a 12-year-old boy showing K-complex in a referential montage with Cz. Note the typical morphology shown by this montage.

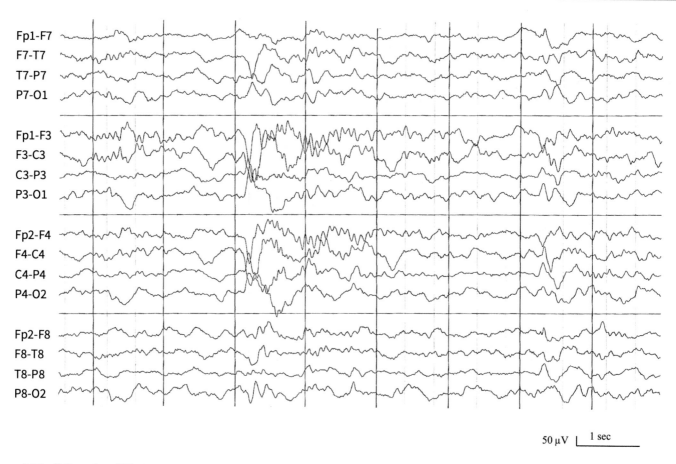

Fp1-F7
F7-T7
T7-P7
P7-O1

Fp1-F3
F3-C3
C3-P3
P3-O1

Fp2-F4
F4-C4
C4-P4
P4-O2

Fp2-F8
F8-T8
T8-P8
P8-O2

50 μV　　1 sec

Figure 7.20　K-Complex. EEG of a 14-year-old boy showing a vertex wave followed by sleep spindles (K-complex).

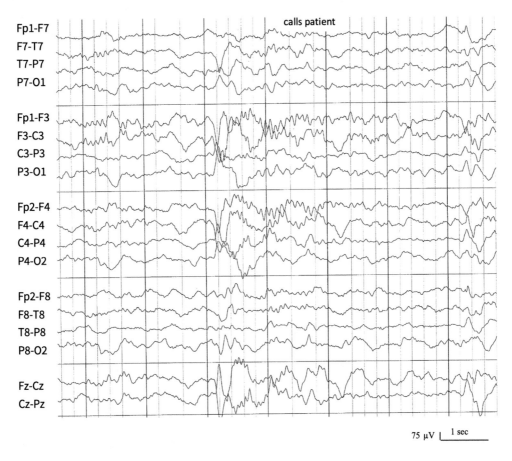

calls patient

Figure 7.21 K-Complex. EEG of a 12-year-old boy showing a vertex wave followed by sleep spindles (K-complex) triggered by calling the patient. K-complex can occur spontaneously or after a sudden stimulus.

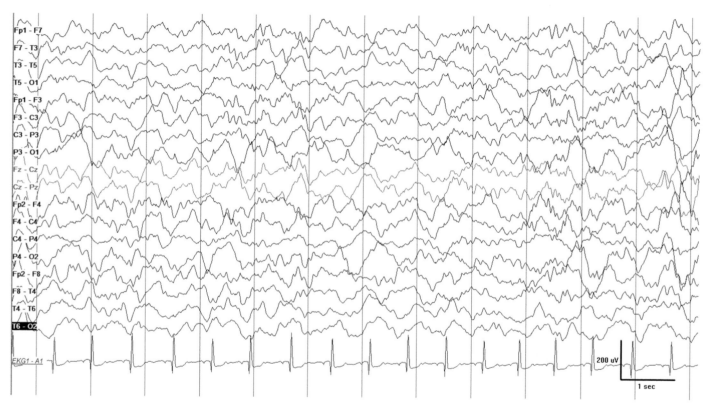

Figure 7.22 N3 sleep (deep sleep, formerly called slow-wave sleep). EEG during sleep showing diffuse delta waves.

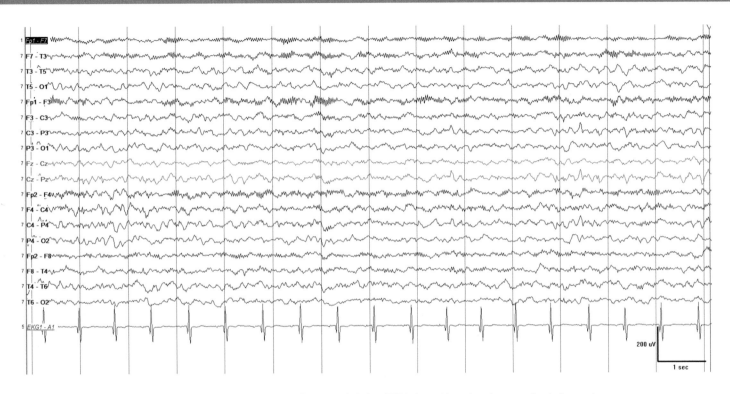

Figure 7.23   REM sleep. EEG showing fast rhythms (alpha frequency) during REM sleep. Note the absence of spindles and v-waves.

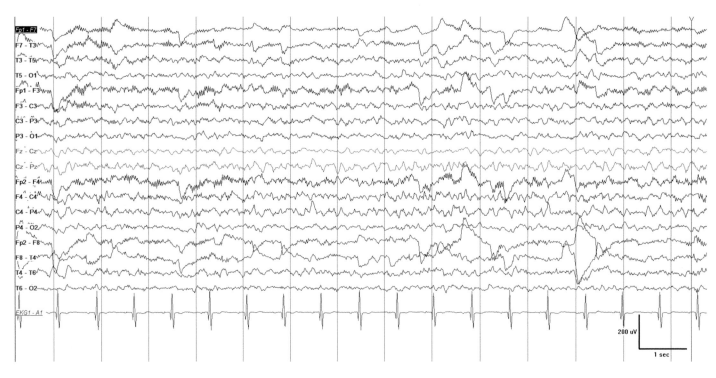

Figure 7.24   REM sleep. EEG showing fast rhythms (alpha frequency) during REM sleep. Note lateral eye-movement artifacts in the anterior channels (rapid eye movements) and the absence of spindles and v-waves.

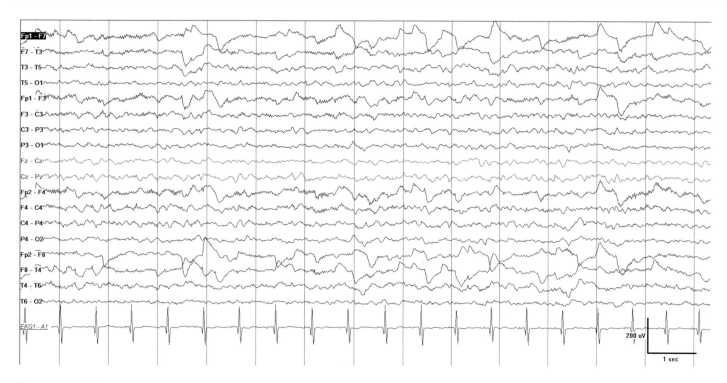

Figure 7.25 REM sleep. EEG showing fast rhythms (alpha frequency) during REM sleep. Note lateral eye-movement artifacts in the anterior channels (rapid eye movements) and the absence of spindles and v-waves.

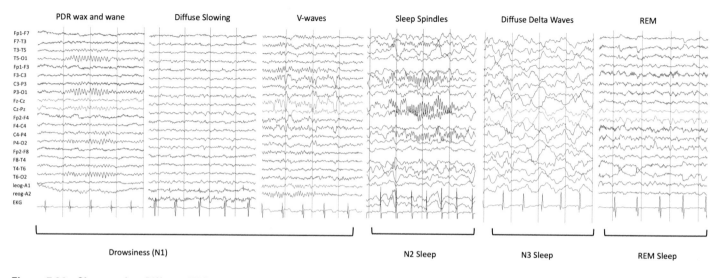

Figure 7.26   Sleep cycles. Different EEG epochs showing the characteristics of each sleep stage (PDR: Posterior dominant rhythm).

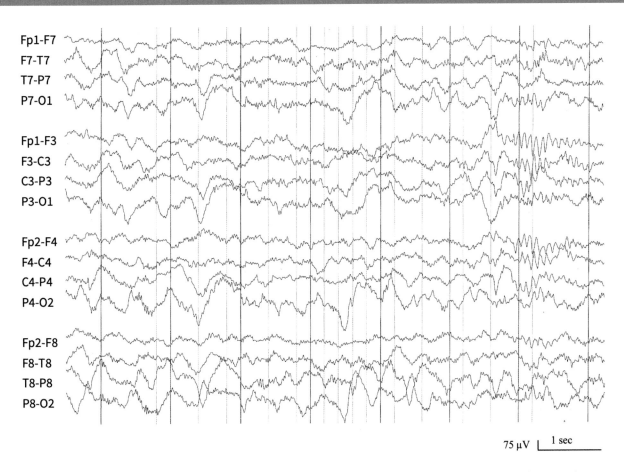

Figure 7.27 Cone waves. EEG of a 2-year-old boy during sleep showing bilateral, high-voltage, cone-shaped occipital delta waves (cone waves). Note synchronous sleep spindles in the last 2 seconds of this sample.

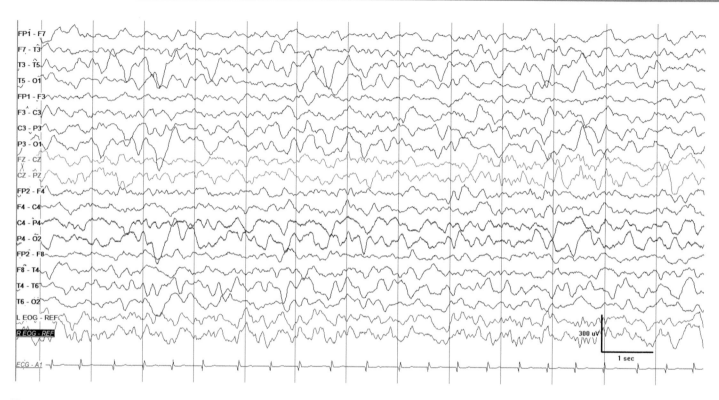

Figure 7.28   Cone waves. EEG of a 15-month-old boy during sleep showing bilateral, high-voltage, cone-shaped occipital delta waves (cone waves).

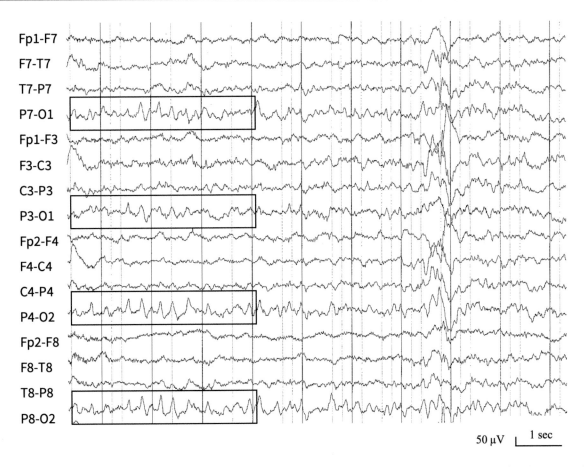

50 µV |__ 1 sec

Figure 7.29   Positive occipital sharp transients of sleep (POSTS). EEG of a 14-year-old girl during sleep showing positive sharp waves in the occipital region (box). This is a normal variant that is not associated with increased risk for seizures.

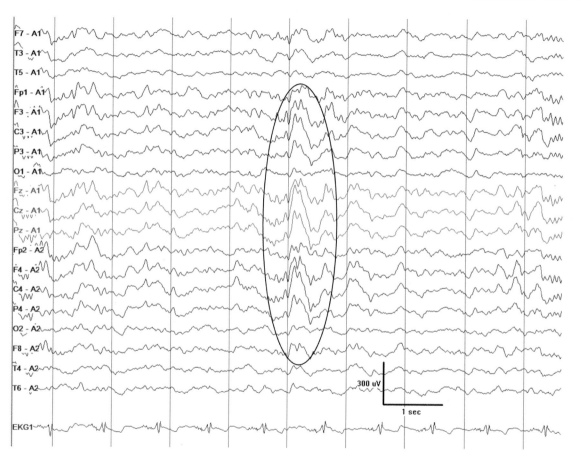

Figure 7.30 Mitten. Sleep EEG showing sharply contoured high-amplitude wave preceded by a small spike of lower amplitude ("thumb of the mitten").

REFERENCES

Amzica F, Steriade M. The K-Complex: Its Slow (<1 Hz) Rhythmicity and Relation to Delta Wavas. Neurology 1997;49:952–59.

Davis KF, Parker KP, Montgomery GL. Sleep in Infants and Young Children: Part One—Normal Sleep. J Pedia Health Care 2004;18:65–71.

Gibbs EL, Gibbs FA. Extreme Spindles. Correlation of Electroencephalographic Sleep Pattern with Mental Retardation. Science 1962;138:1106–07.

Hughes JR. EEG in Clinical Practice. 2nd Ed. Newton: Butterworth-Heinemann; 1994.

Montenegro MA, Cendes F, Guerreiro MM, Guerreiro CAM. EEG na Pratica Clinica. Rio de Janeiro: Thieme-Reventer; 2022.

Riviello JJ Jr, Nordli DR Jr, Niedermeyer E. Normal EEG and Sleep: Infants and Adolescents. In: Schomer, DL, da Silva, FHL (Eds). Niedermeyer's Electroencephalography: Basic Principles, Clinical Applications, and Related Fields, 6th Ed. Philadelphia: Lippincott Williams & Wilkins; 2011. p. 321–57.

CHAPTER 8

Non-epileptiform abnormalities

Brittany Sprigg, MD

Maria Augusta Montenegro, MD, PhD

Non-epileptiform abnormalities are associated with transitory or permanent dysfunction but not with an increased risk of seizures. There are several types of non-epileptiform abnormalities:

- Slowing
- Asymmetry
- Asynchrony
- Absence of physiological sleep elements
- Periodic discharges
- Excessive beta

As opposed to what is seen in adult EEG recordings, slow waves in childhood can be normal on several occasions. The most common situations are:

a. Posterior dominant rhythm varies according to the patient's age, and as the brain matures, it becomes faster. A rudimentary posterior dominant rhyythm starts to develop at 2 to 3 months old, and by 3 to 4 months, it shows some reactivity to eye opening and closure (**Figure 8.1**). At the same age, faster activity in central regions appears and the anterior-posterior gradient starts to develop (Riviello *et al.*, 2011). Most children will have a posterior dominant rhythm of 8 Hz at 3 years old. Until the age of 8, however, a slower frequency may be seen without it being considered abnormal (**Table 8.1**).

b. Posterior slow waves of youth are square-shaped delta waves at the posterior regions (same region of the posterior dominant rhythm), bilateral or unilateral. They are usually seen from the second half of the first decade until adolescence (**Figure 8.2**). Slow waves of youth are seen with eyes closed and are blocked by eye-opening.

DOI: 10.1201/b23339-8

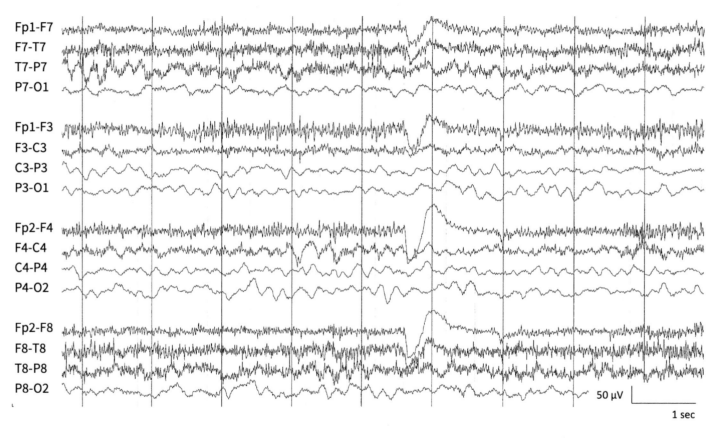

Figure 8.1 Normal background. EEG of a 4-month-old patient during wakefulness showing a normal background characterized by a mixture of theta and delta waves and a posterior dominant rhythm of 4–5 Hz.

Table 8.1   Posterior dominant rhythm (PDR) according to each age

Age	Most common PDR	Minimum PDR required
1 year old	6	5
2 years old	7	5
3 years old	8	6
5 years old	9	7
8 years old	9	8
10 years old	10	8

c. Hypnagogic hypersynchrony is characterized by high-amplitude sinusoidal theta waves seen during drowsiness (**Figures 8.3** and **8.4**). It appears during the first year of life and persists throughout the first decade and early teenage years. Hypnopompic hypersynchrony (or arousal reaction) has the same characteristics as hypnagogic hypersynchrony but is seen upon arousal. Both are rare in adults.

d. Hyperventilation can trigger bilateral and synchronous slowing, which can be exuberant (high amplitude and delta frequency) in younger patients (**Figure 8.5**). In children, the slowing may predominate posteriorly and in adolescents it is more prominent anteriorly (Fisch, 1991; Goldberg & Strauss, 1959). Despite the anteroposterior predominance according to age group, the distribution of slow waves should be diffuse, without focal or persistent lateralization. The slowing should disappear and return to the baseline frequency one minute after the end of hyperventilation. Low blood glucose may exacerbate the slowing.

Although theta and delta waves are normal in the awake EEG recording of very young children, diffuse, very frequent, or continuous theta and delta waves should be considered abnormal in older children. Diffuse background slowing is associated with diffuse subcortical dysfunction (**Figures 8.6–8.10**). During coma, the EEG is characterized by diffuse slowing, with a good correlation between wave frequency and severity of symptoms (slower recordings correlate with more severe symptoms; **Figure 8.10**). Sleep transients (spindles, v-waves, and K complex) may also be absent (**Figures 8.11** and **8.12**).

The unilateral absence of posterior dominant rhythm reactivity to eye-opening and closure (Bancaud phenomenon) is associated with ipsilateral structural lesion in the posterior region.

The amplitude of the posterior dominant rhythm varies from individual to individual, and even in the same patient (Chang *et al.*, 2011). In adults, the posterior dominant rhythm has an amplitude between 40 and 50 μV, but higher amplitudes are frequently seen in younger patients. Mild posterior dominant rhythm asymmetry is considered normal, with higher amplitude seen in the non-dominant hemisphere. Although amplitude asymmetry higher than 50% (**Figure 8.13**) may represent an abnormal finding, it should be carefully evaluated (Markand, 1990) because one of the most common reasons for amplitude asymmetry is different distances between electrodes from homologous areas.

In addition to the amplitude of the waves, asymmetry also applies to wave frequency: a) Mild asymmetry: Asymmetry <50% in amplitude on referential montage or frequency 0.5–1 Hz; b) Marked asymmetry: Asymmetry ≥50% in voltage or

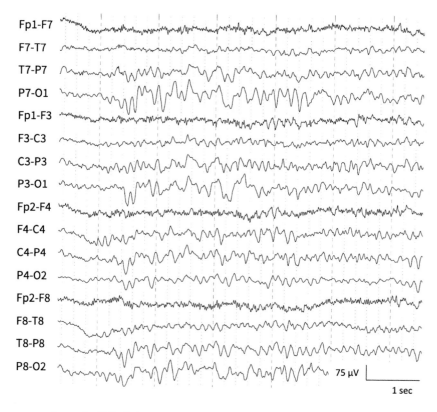

Figure 8.2   Posterior slow waves of youth. EEG during wakefulness of a 12-year-old boy showing square-shaped delta waves in the posterior regions (seconds 2 to 4, in the same region of the posterior dominant rhythm). Slow waves of youth can be unilateral or bilateral.

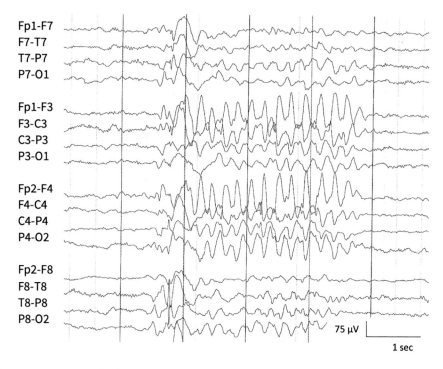

Figure 8.3   Hypnagogic hypersynchrony. EEG of a 5-year-old boy showing high-amplitude diffuse sinusoidal theta waves during drowsiness.

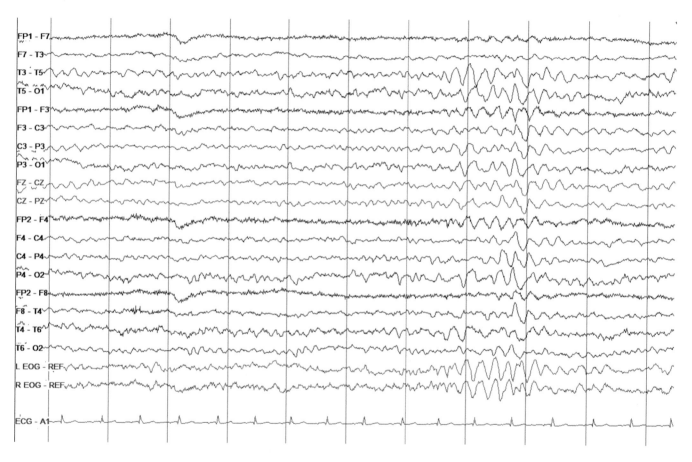

Figure 8.4 Hypnagogic hypersynchrony. EEG showing high-amplitude diffuse medium/high-amplitude sinusoidal theta waves during drowsiness.

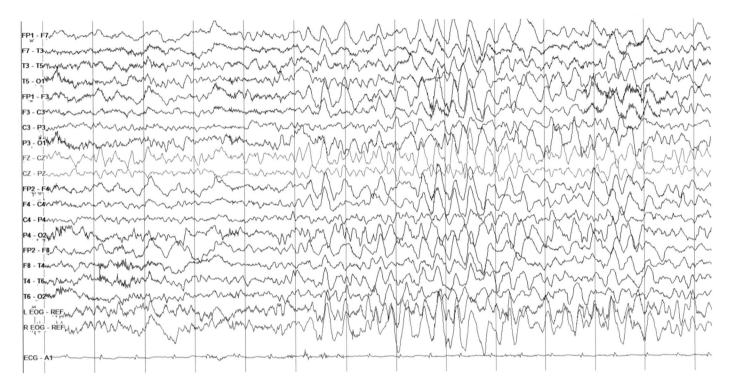

Figure 8.5   Hyperventilation. EEG showing diffuse high-amplitude slow waves triggered by hyperventilation. The slowing is usually gradual and can reach impressive levels, characterized by diffuse high-amplitude delta waves.

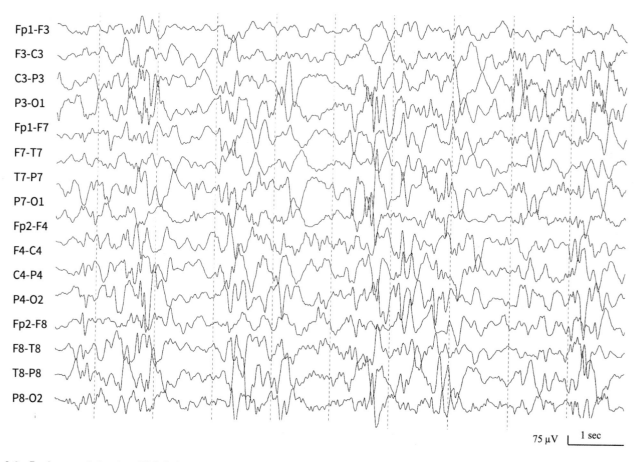

75 μV | 1 sec

Figure 8.6 Background slowing. EEG during sleep showing hypsarrhythmia, characterized by disorganized background with diffuse theta and delta waves and absence of normal sleep transients (sleep spindles, v-waves, K-complex). Also note the multifocal spikes and sharp waves.

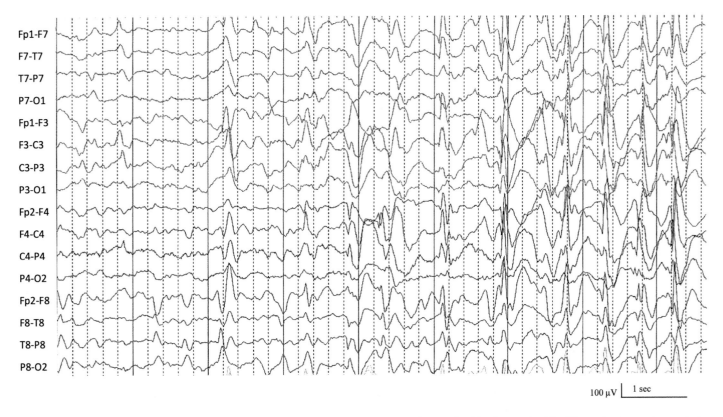

100 µV | 1 sec

Figure 8.7 Diffuse background slowing. EEG during wakefulness showing poorly organized background with diffuse slowing and no anterior-posterior gradient. Also note the generalized spike-wave complexes (<2.5 Hz), associated with Lennox-Gastaut syndrome.

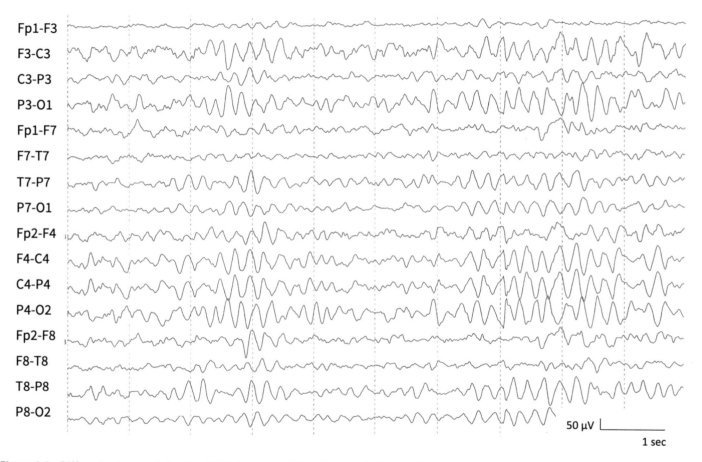

Figure 8.8   Diffuse background slowing. EEG of a 4-year-old boy during wakefulness showing diffuse background slowing characterized by monomorphic biparietal theta rhythm (4–7 Hz). This patient has epilepsy with myoclonic atonic seizures (Doose syndrome).

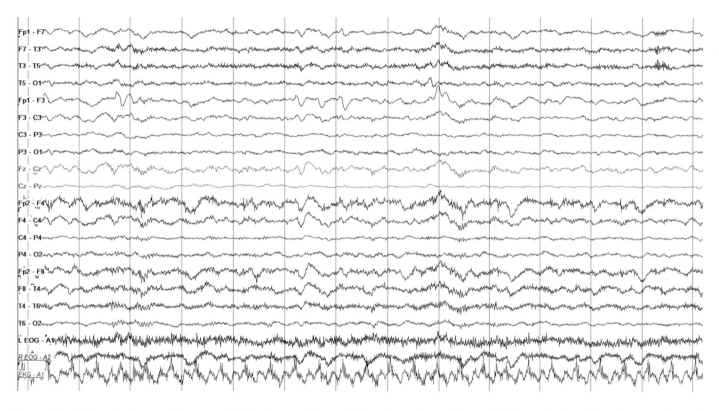

Figure 8.9   Diffuse background slowing. EEG of a 9-year-old boy with Dravet syndrome during wakefulness showing diffuse background slowing characterized by medium-amplitude diffuse theta and delta range waves. No clear anterior to posterior gradient or posterior dominant rhythm can be identified.

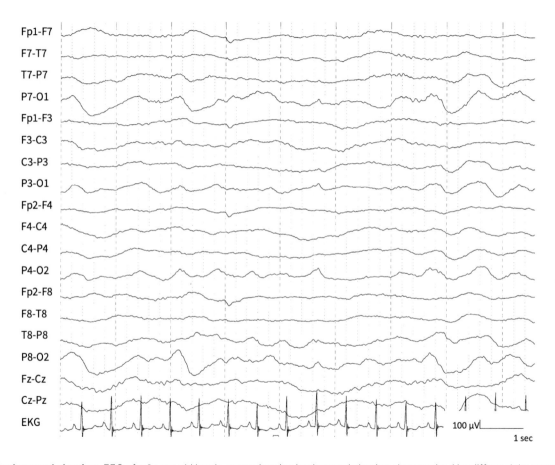

Figure 8.10   Background slowing. EEG of a 9-year-old boy in coma showing background slowing characterized by diffuse delta waves.

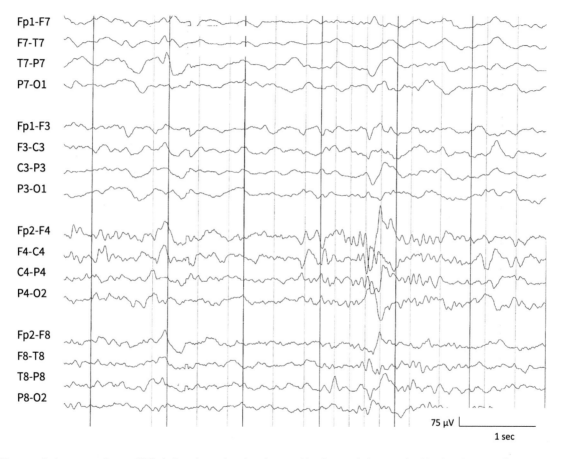

Figure 8.11   Abnormal sleep transients. EEG during sleep showing abnormal background characterized by the absence of sleep transients in the left hemisphere in a patient with a left hemisphere tumor.

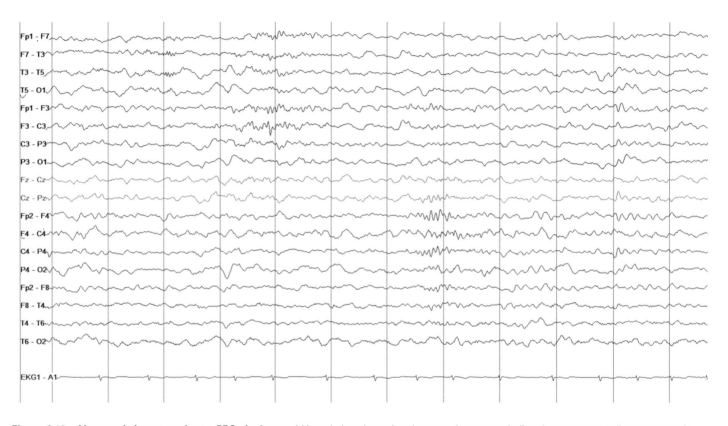

Figure 8.12   Abnormal sleep transients. EEG of a 2-year-old boy during sleep showing asynchronous spindles due to corpus callosum agenesis.

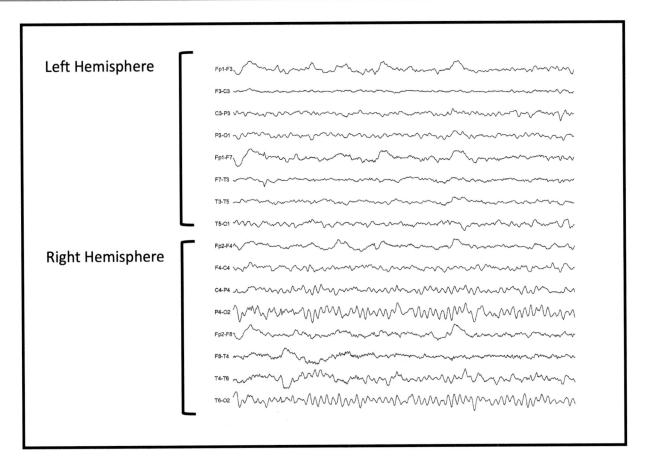

Figure 8.13   Amplitude asymmetry. EEG showing a posterior dominant rhythm with higher amplitude in the right hemisphere.

>1 Hz in frequency (**Figure 8.14**; Hirsch et al., 2021). Asymmetry can also be caused by extracerebral conditions, and increased amplitude is associated with skull defect (breach rhythm; **Figure 8.15**). Decreased amplitude might be due to blood (caput succedaneum, cephalohematoma, and epidural or subdural hematomas) or cerebral spinal fluid collections between the brain and electrodes (**Figure 8.16**).

Other types of non-epileptiform abnormalities include:

a. Intermittent slowing is characterized by focal or diffuse polymorphic theta/delta (usually theta) waves for a few seconds. This is non-specific but can be associated with focal or diffuse cortical dysfunction (**Figures 8.17–8.19**).

b. Continuous focal slowing is characterized by focal continuous (or nearly continuous) polymorphic theta or delta waves. It is frequently associated with subcortical dysfunction, mostly due to an underlying structural lesion (**Figures 8.20** and **8.21**).

c. Rhythmic delta activity (previously called intermittent rhythmic delta activity: IRDA) is characterized by monomorphic rhythmic delta waves, usually over one cerebral region (**Figures 8.22–8.25**). It should not be used for seizure lateralization (even if unilateral), except if it is in the temporal region (where it is considered equivalent to epileptiform activity and can be used to lateralize a possible epileptic focus; Gambardella et al., 1995). Rhythmic delta activity in the occipital region of patients with absence epilepsy is usually asynchronous, attenuated by eye-opening and triggered by hyperventilation. It is more frequent in younger patients and is associated with childhood absence epilepsy. It may occur in patients with juvenile absence epilepsy, but it is uncommon. In children with absence epilepsy, it correlates with a more favorable prognosis with comparatively rare occurrence of generalized tonic-clonic seizures (Guilhoto et al., 2006).

d. Medication can cause diffuse slowing, and the most common drugs associated with it are anesthetics, sedatives, and antiseizure medications (**Figures 8.26** and **8.27**).

e. Periodic discharges with triphasic morphology are associated with metabolic encephalopathy, classically especially due to hepatic or renal failure (**Figures 8.28** and **8.29**).

f. Periodic discharges are uniform wave repetitions for at least six cycles, with a regular interval between them. It is classified as generalized, lateralized, or bilateral independent (Hirsch et al., 2021). Periodic discharges are seen in herpes simplex type 1 encephalitis, subacute sclerosing panencephalitis, medications (propofol, thiopental, etc.), Creutzfeldt-Jakob disease, etc. Lateralized periodic discharges (LPDs; formerly called PLEDs: periodic lateralized epileptiform discharges) are associated with subacute cortical/subcortical injury and are not specific for herpes simples virus type 1 encephalitis. It reflects subacute focal structural or functional impairment, whether it is from a lesion or an acute infarct (**Figures 8.30–8.32**).

g. Excessive fast activity is a non-specific finding and is usually associated with the use of benzodiazepines or barbiturates (**Figure 8.33**).

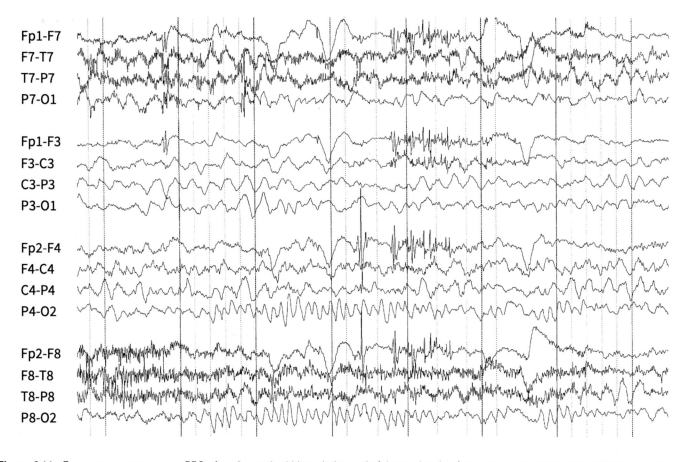

Figure 8.14 Frequency asymmetry. EEG of an 8-month-old boy during wakefulness showing frequency asymmetry characterized by continuous slow waves (4–5 Hz) in the left hemisphere. Note the well-developed 9 Hz posterior dominant rhythm in the right hemisphere.

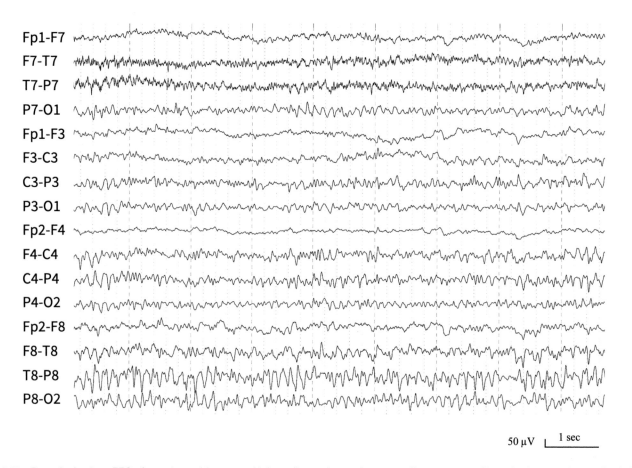

50 μV ⌊ 1 sec

Figure 8.15　Breach rhythm. EEG of a patient with temporal lobe epilepsy that underwent epilepsy surgery. Note the increase in amplitude in right temporoparietal region (under the skull defect).

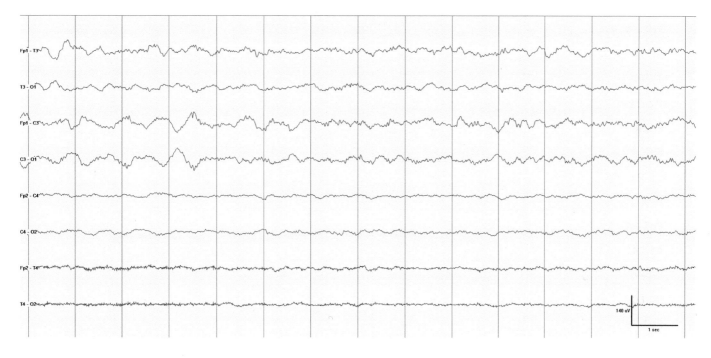

Figure 8.16   Asymmetry. EEG of a 4 month-old baby showing inter-hemispheric asymmetry due to a subdural hematoma in the right hemisphere.

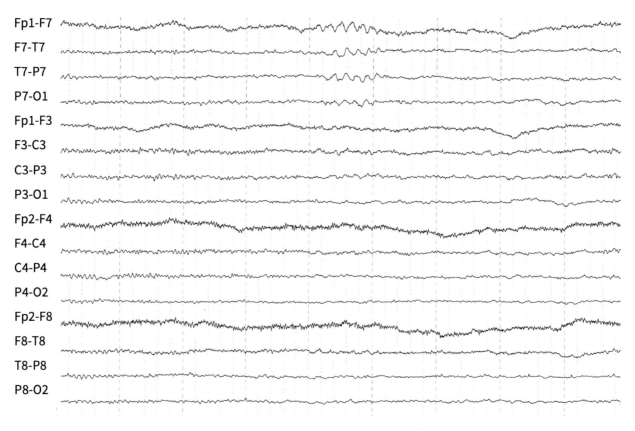

Figure 8.17 Intermittent focal slowing. EEG of a 16-year-old patient with temporal lobe epilepsy showing intermittent polymorphic theta range waves in the left temporal region.

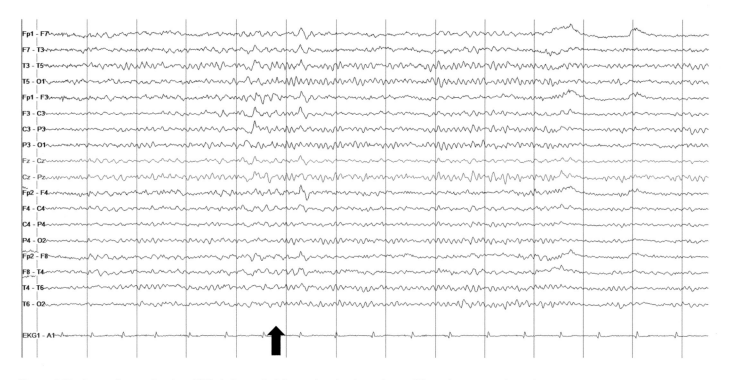

Figure 8.18 Intermittent slowing. EEG during wakefulness showing intermittent diffuse theta waves (arrow).

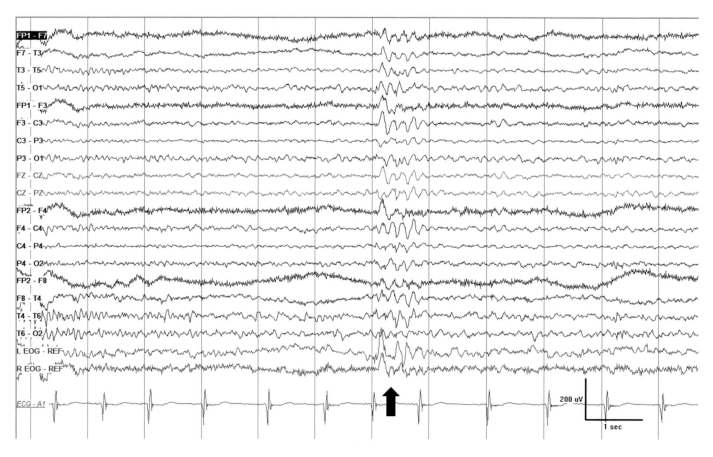

Figure 8.19   Intermittent slowing. EEG during wakefulness showing intermittent diffuse theta waves (arrow).

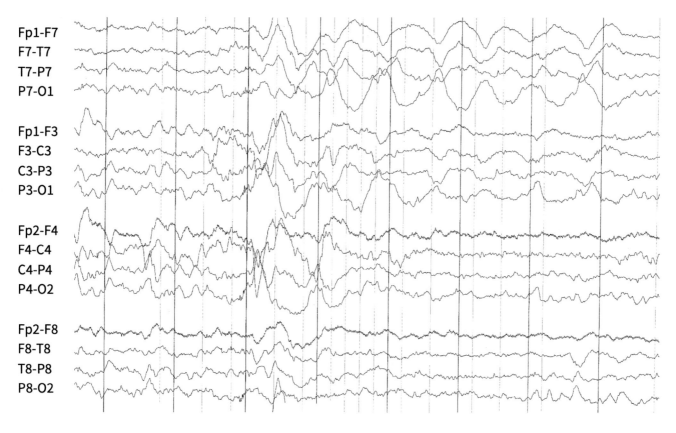

Figure 8.20   Focal slowing. EEG during sleep showing very frequent, almost continuous, runs of sharply contoured delta waves over the left hemisphere. Also note that the sleep elements are better formed in the right hemisphere. This finding was associated with a structural lesion (tumor) in the left hemisphere.

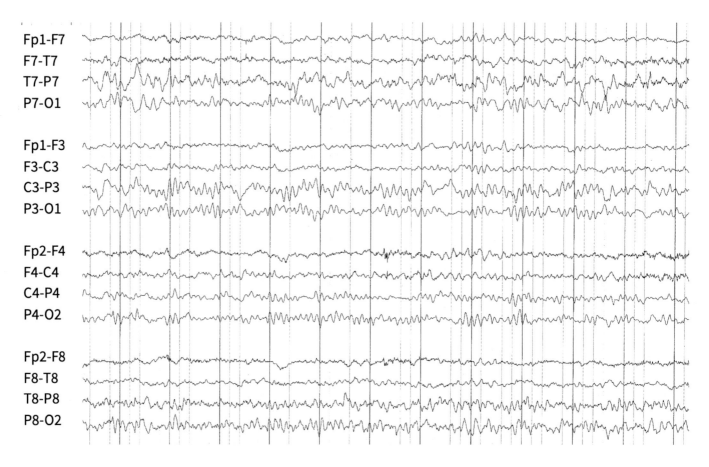

Figure 8.21 Focal slowing. EEG during wakefulness showing very frequent, almost continuous slowing in the left posterior quadrant.

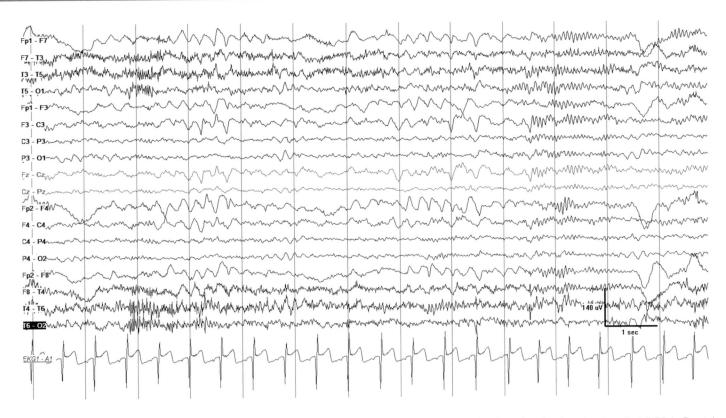

Figure 8.22 Rhythmic delta activity. EEG showing high-amplitude rhythmic delta activity in the frontal region (previously called FIRDA: Frontal intermittent rhythmic delta activity), more evident in the right hemisphere.

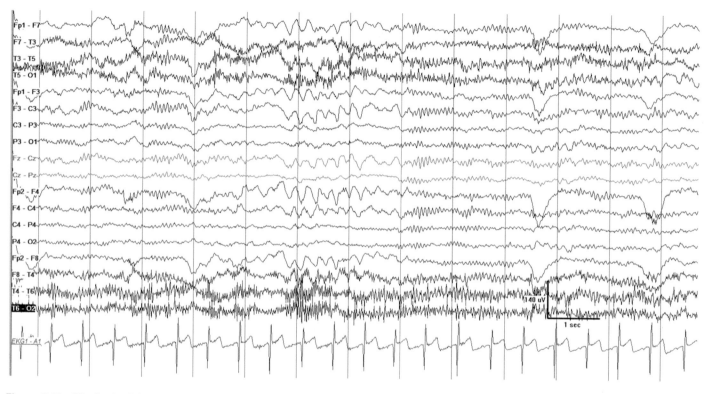

Figure 8.23 Rhythmic delta activity. EEG showing high-amplitude rhythmic delta activity in the frontal region (previously called FIRDA: Frontal intermittent rhythmic delta activity), more evident in the right hemisphere.

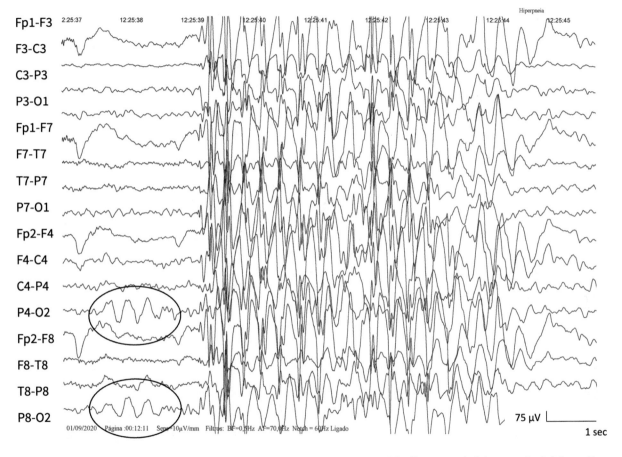

Figure 8.24   Childhood absence epilepsy. EEG showing right occipital rhythmic delta activity (first second of the recording), followed by generalized regular 3 Hz spike-wave complexes for 5 seconds.

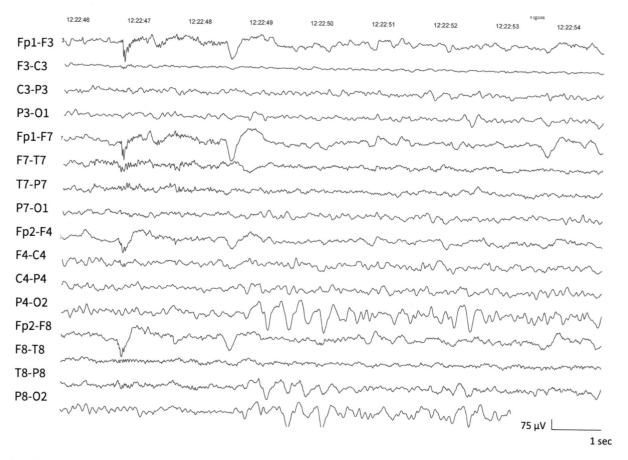

Figure 8.25   Childhood absence epilepsy. EEG showing right occipital rhythmic delta activity. This finding in children with childhood absence epilepsy may correlate with more favorable prognosis (rare occurrence of GTCs).

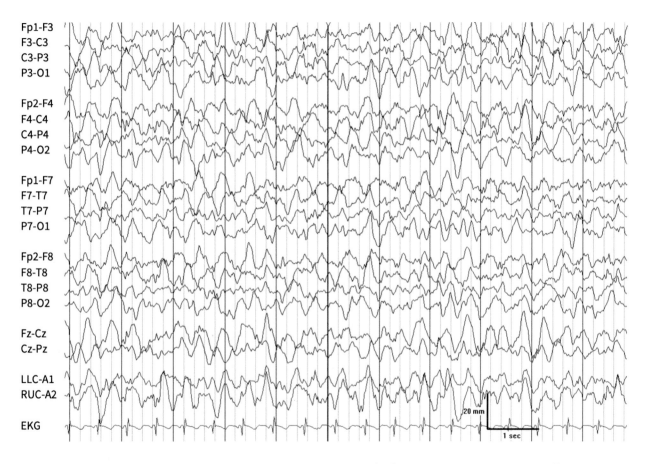

Figure 8.26   Background slowing due to medication. EEG during sedation (propofol) for a medical procedure showing diffuse high-amplitude slow waves.

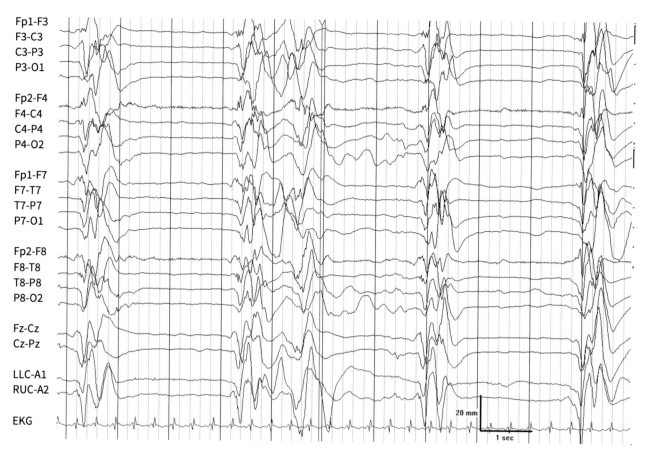

Figure 8.27 Burst suppression due to medication. EEG during sedation for medical procedure showing diffuse high-amplitude sharp and slow waves followed by diffuse voltage attenuation. This is the same patient from the previous figure, now with a higher dose of propofol.

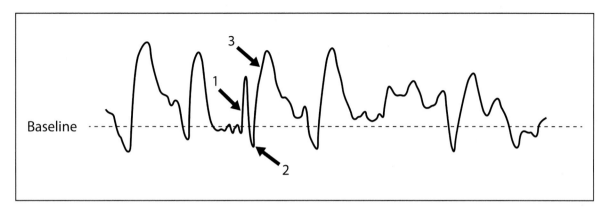

Figure 8.28   How to measure the number of wave phases. Each phase (numbered in the figure) must be above or below the baseline (the typical discharge must cross the baseline two times to be considered a triphasic wave).

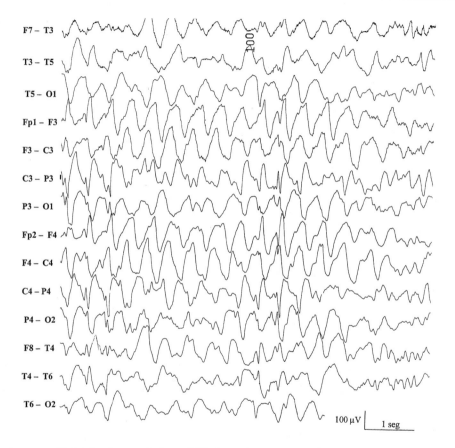

Figure 8.29   Periodic discharges with triphasic morphology. EEG of a patient with metabolic encephalopathy due to hepatic failure showing diffuse periodic discharges with triphasic morphology. (Reproduced from Montenegro *et al.*, 2022, with permission.)

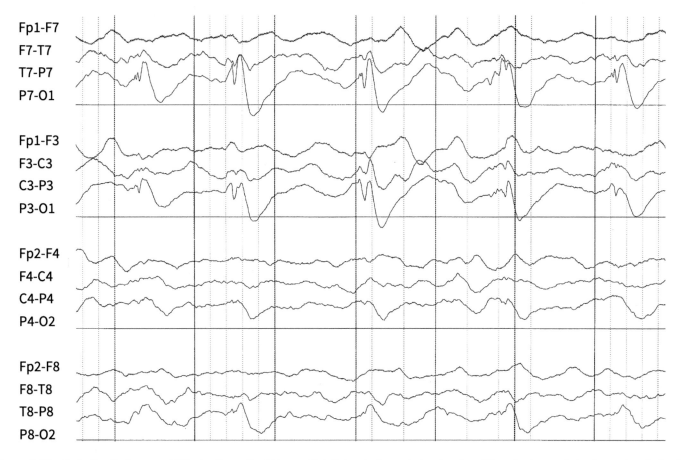

Figure 8.30   Periodic discharges. EEG of a 3-month-old boy with left hemisphere stroke showing diffuse background slowing and periodic discharges in the left parieto-occipital region.

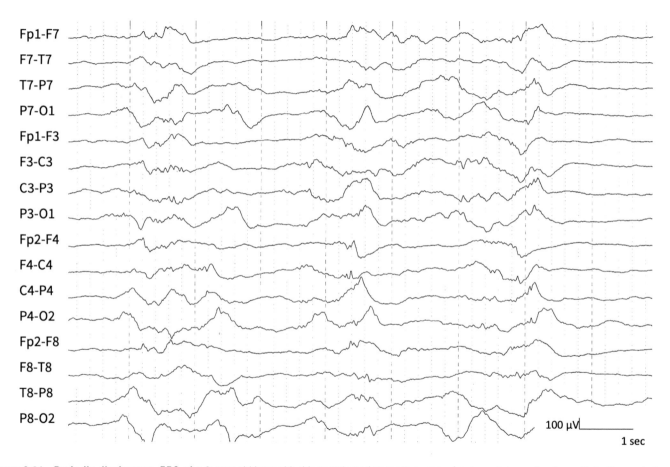

Figure 8.31   Periodic discharges. EEG of a 9-year-old boy with thiopental used to treat super refractory status epilepticus. Note the periodic discharges characterized by generalized sharp waves followed by diffuse attenuation of the voltage.

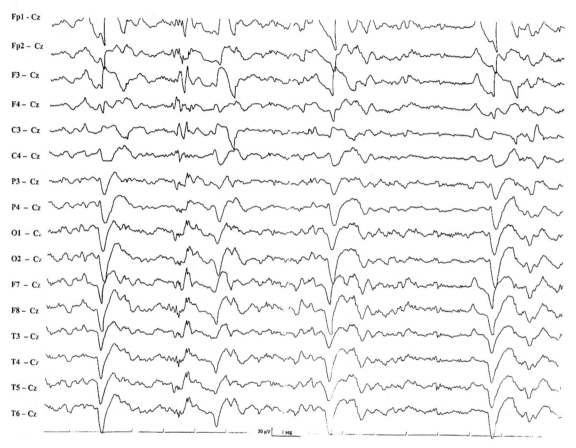

Figure 8.32 Periodic discharges. EEG during wakefulness of a 7-year-old boy with subacute sclerosis panencephalitis showing high-amplitude sharply contoured periodic discharges. (Radermecker complex; reproduced from Montenegro *et al.*, 2022, with permission.)

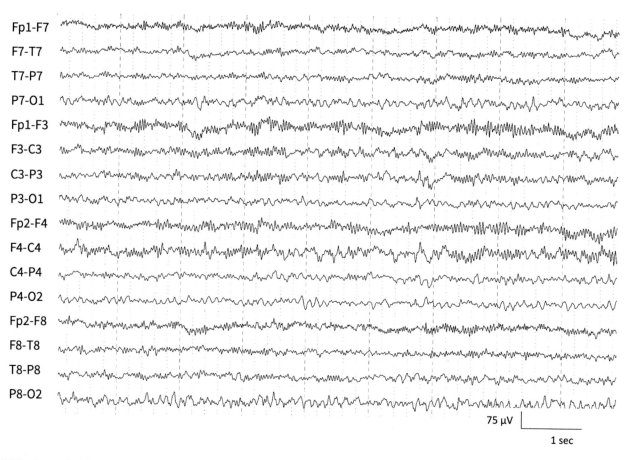

Figure 8.33 Excessive beta activity. EEG during wakefulness showing excessive beta activity in a patient on a high dose of benzodiazepine (clobazam).

REFERENCES

Chang BS, Schomer DL, Niedermeyer E. Normal EEG and Sleep: Adults and Elderly. In: Schomer, DL, da Silva, FHL (Eds). Niedermeyer's Electroencephalography: Basic Principles, Clinical Applications, and Related Fields, 6th Ed. Philadelphia: Lippincott Williams & Wilkins; 2011. p. 358–430.

Fisch BJ. Spehlmann's EEG Primer. 2nd Ed. Amsterdam: Elsevier; 1991.

Gambardella A, Gotman J, Cendes F, Andermann F. Focal Intermittent Delta Activity in Patients with Mesiotemporal Atrophy: A Reliable Marker of the Epileptogenic Focus. Epilepsia 1995;36:122–29.

Goldberg HH, Strauss H. Distribution of Slow Activity Induced by Hyperventilation. Electroencephalogr Clin Neurophysiol 1959;11:615.

Guilhoto LM, Manreza ML, Yacubian EM. Occipital intermittent rhythmic delta activity in absence epilepsy. Arq Neuropsiquiatr 2006 Jun;64(2A):193–97.

Hirsch LJ, Fong MWK, Leitnger M, et al. American Clinical Neurophysiology Society's Standardized Critical Care EEG Terminology: 2021 Version. J Clin Neurophysiol 2021;38:1–29.

Markand OM. Alpha Rhythms. J Clin Neurophysiol 1990;7:163–89.

Montenegro MA, Cendes F, Guerreiro MM, Guerreiro CAM. EEG na Pratica Clinica. Rio de Janeiro: Thieme-Revinter; 2022.

Riviello JJ Jr, Nordli DR Jr, Niedermeyer E. Normal EEG and Sleep: Infants and Adolescents. In: Schomer, DL, da Silva, FHL (Eds). Niedermeyer's Electroencephalography: Basic Principles, Clinical Applications, and Related Fields, 6th Ed. Philadelphia: Lippincott Williams & Wilkins; 2011. p. 321–57.

CHAPTER 9

Focal epilepsy syndromes

Shifteh Sattar, MD

Maria Augusta Montenegro, MD, PhD

Focal epilepsy has several revised terminologies. Self-limited is the term currently used to substitute the previously used terms "benign" and "idiopathic" as descriptors of childhood epilepsies (Berg *et al.*, 2010). The revision was deemed necessary given the possible cognitive and psychosocial consequences of some childhood epilepsy syndromes, sometimes neglected once seizure freedom is achieved. Self-limited epilepsy syndromes are characterized by the following (Specchio *et al.*, 2022):

- Age-dependent occurrence, specific for each syndrome.
- No significant structural lesion of the brain.
- Birth, neonatal, and antecedent history is usually unremarkable.
- Cognition and neurological examination are typically normal.

- Remission usually occurs by adolescence.
- Seizures are easily controlled by antiseizure medication (in most cases, but not all patients).
- Genetic predisposition for the EEG trait.
- Classical seizure semiology for each syndrome.
- Seizures are focal motor or sensory with or without impaired awareness and may evolve to bilateral tonic-clonic seizures.
- Specific EEG features: Epileptiform discharges with distinctive morphology and location (depending on the epilepsy syndrome), often activated with sleep.
- EEG has a normal background.

DOI: 10.1201/b23339-9

The EEG characteristics of the most common childhood epilepsy syndromes are described below.

Self-Limited (Familial) Infantile Epilepsy (SeLIE)

- Age: Usually between 18 and 36 months old.
- Seizure type: Focal seizures characterized by behavioral arrest, impaired awareness, automatisms, head and/or eye version, and clonic movements.
- Former names: Benign familial (and non-familial) infantile seizures.
- EEG findings: Normal background, usually no interictal discharges.

Self-Limited Epilepsy with Centrotemporal Spikes (SeLECTS)

- Age: Usually between 3 and 14 years old.
- Seizure type: Seizures are characterized by unilateral sensory (numbness or paresthesia of face, mouth, tongue) and/or motor (hemifacial tonic or clonic movements) symptoms, hypersalivation, speech arrest (dysarthria or anarthria).
- Bilateral tonic-clonic seizures may occur, mostly at sleep onset or in the early morning.
- Former names: Rolandic epilepsy, childhood epilepsy with centrotemporal spikes, idiopathic or benign centrotemporal epilepsy.
- EEG findings: Normal background and high-amplitude diphasic spike or sharp-and-slow waves (100–300 μV), isolated or in clusters, unilateral or bilateral, synchronous, or independent, at the centrotemporal regions (T5, T6, C3, C4). The discharges may occur outside the centrotemporal region, at the frontal or parietal electrodes. The sharp-slow waves are usually activated by drowsiness or sleep, and in one third of the patients, the EEG will show sharp-slow waves only during sleep. At the referential montage, the epileptiform discharges are frequently shown as a horizontal (transverse) dipole, because the EEG registers both the negative and positive ends to the dipole (because the discharge is usually deep in the sulci), which will be seen as a positive polarity wave (sharp wave "downward') at the anterior electrodes and as a negative polarity wave (sharp wave "upward") at the more posterior electrodes. Although the background is normal, when the spike or sharp-slow waves occur very frequently, there may be focal slowing in the same region (pseudo slowing; Holmes, 1993)
- Hyperventilation and photic stimulation do not have any impact on the recording (**Figures 9.1–9.8**).
- Atypical SeLECTS: A rare entity characterized by cognitive impairment, behavioral abnormalities, and/or continuous spike-and-wave during slow sleep. Language regression can also occur (Fejerman et al., 2000). Due to significant overlap of symptoms among the atypical evolution of Rolandic epilepsy, Landau-Kleffner syndrome, and electrographic status epilepticus of sleep/continuous spike-wave during sleep (ESES/CSWS), they are now classified as a single entity called Developmental Encephalopathy with Spike and Wave Activation during Sleep (Specchio et al., 2022).

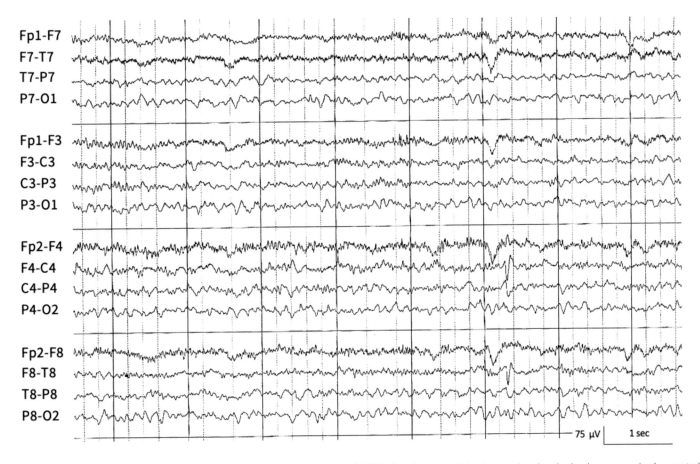

Figure 9.1   Self-limited epilepsy with centrotemporal spikes (awake). EEG showing normal background and a single sharp wave in the central region (C4).

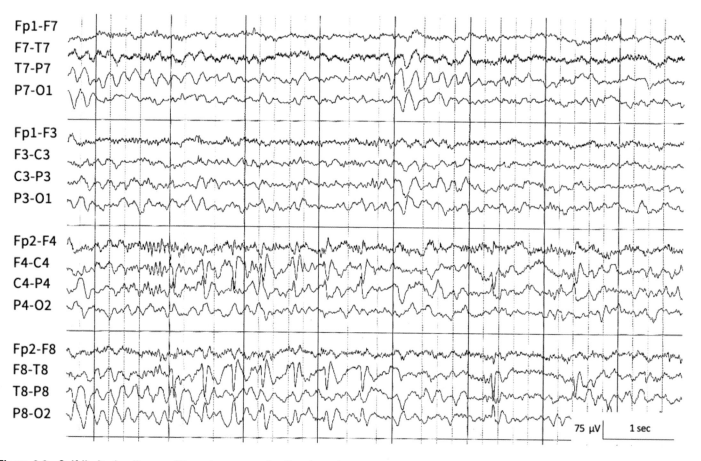

Figure 9.2   Self-limited epilepsy with centrotemporal spikes (sleep). EEG showing normal background during sleep and several sharp waves in the centrotemporal region. This is the same patient from **Figure 9.1**, same day of recording, note the sleep activation of the discharges.

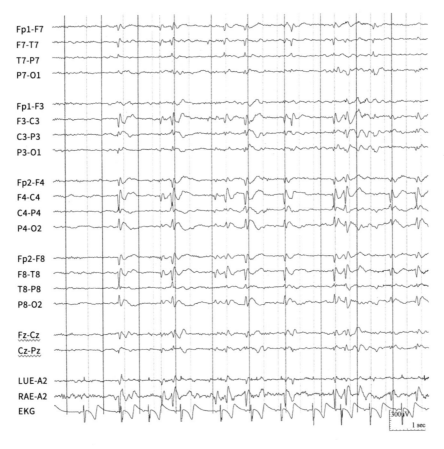

Figure 9.3   Self-limited epilepsy with centrotemporal spikes (awake). Bipolar montage showing normal background and several sharp waves in the centrotemporal region, with more prominent phase reversal in C4 and T8.

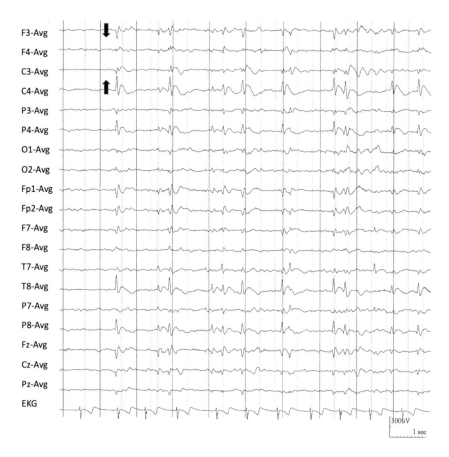

Figure 9.4 Self-limited epilepsy with centrotemporal spikes (awake). Same patient from the previous figure, now on a referential montage showing normal background and several sharp waves in the centrotemporal region, with higher amplitude in C4 and T8. Note the horizontal dipole where the frontal electrodes (arrow down) show a shift in the polarity when compared with the more posterior electrodes (arrow up).

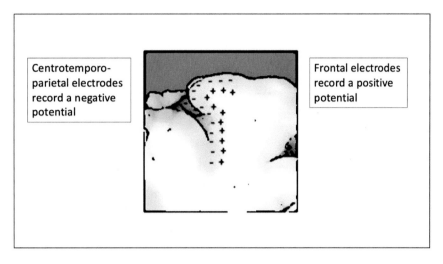

Figure 9.5 Horizontal dipole. Referential montages enable the recording of horizontal dipoles, showing the negative (posterior electrodes) and positive (anterior electrodes, usually frontal areas) voltage of the dipole. It occurs because the focus is deep in the sulci, with neurons parallel to the scalp. It will be seen as a positive polarity wave (sharp wave "downward") at the anterior electrodes and as a negative polarity wave (sharp wave "upward") at the more posterior electrodes.

Self-Limited Epilepsy with Autonomic Seizures (SeLEAS)

- Age: Usually between 1 and 14 years old (most frequently 2–6 years old).

- Seizure type: Most seizures occur during sleep and are characterized by focal autonomic seizures associated with eye or head deviation with or without impaired awareness. Vomiting is the most common autonomic feature, but other autonomic symptoms (pupillary abnormalities, pallor, cyanosis, changes in body temperature, etc.) may occur.

- Status epilepticus is common.

- Former names: Panayiotopoulos syndrome.

- EEG findings: Normal background with focal spikes/sharp waves followed by slow waves that may involve any region of the brain, even with multi-focal involvement. The morphology of the discharges are similar to the discharges seen in self-limited epilepsy with centrotemporal spikes. Serial EEGs may show variable localization of the epileptiform abnormalities. The discharges may be activated by sleep and the discharges at the

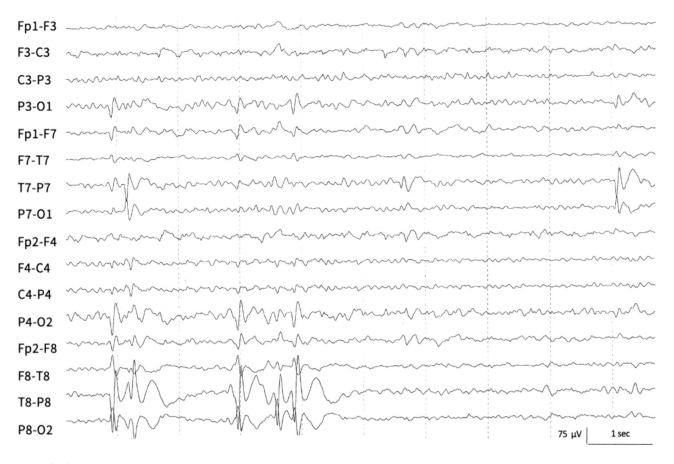

Figure 9.6 Self-limited epilepsy with centrotemporal spikes: Pseudo slowing (awake). EEG showing independent sharp waves followed by slow waves in the right parietal and frontotemporal and left parietal areas. In the right parietal area, the discharges are more prominent and are associated with pseudo slowing.

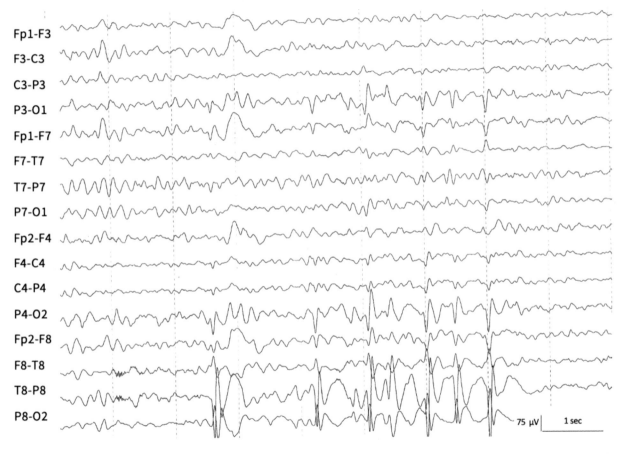

Figure 9.7   Self-limited epilepsy with centrotemporal spikes (awake): Pseudo slowing. EEG showing right parietal sharp waves followed by slow waves. Although the background is normal, when the spike or sharp-and-slow-waves occur very frequently, there may be focal slowing in the region of the spikes (pseudo slowing).

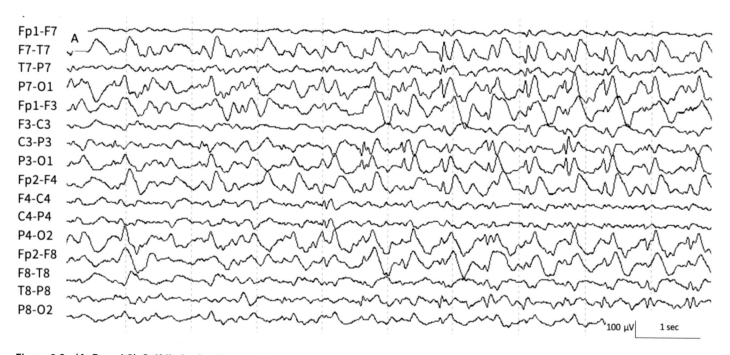

Figure 9.8   (A, B, and C): Self-limited epilepsy with centrotemporal spikes: Ictal. EEG showing a focal seizure in the left fronto-temporo-parietal region, with some degree of involvement of the contralateral homologous regions. During this seizure, the patient experienced clonic movements in the right side of the face for 18 seconds.   *(Continued)*

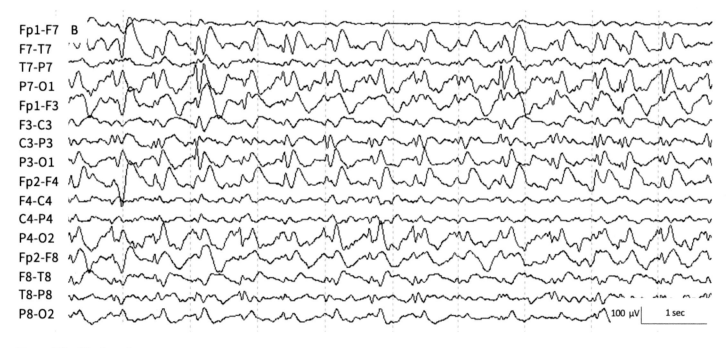

Figure 9.8 *(Continued)*

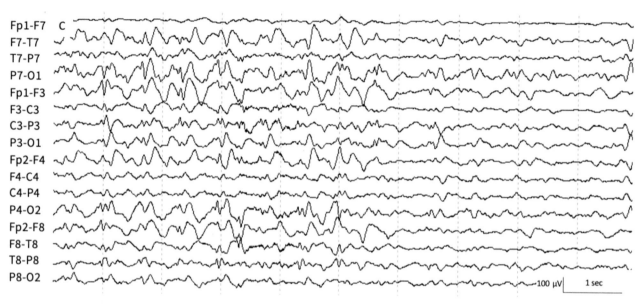

Figure 9.8 *(Continued)*

occipital region might be increased by eye closure and disappear after eye-opening. Hyperventilation and photic stimulation do not have any impact on the recording (**Figures 9.9–9.11**).

Childhood Occipital Visual Epilepsy (COVE)

- Age: Usually between 6 and 15 years old.
- Seizure type: Seizures are characterized by focal visual symptoms for a few seconds to a few minutes. It is frequently followed by bilateral tonic-clonic (or hemi-clonic) seizure. The child

usually describes the visual symptoms as colored small bright lights at the center of the visual field. Headache with migraine like characteristics often occur in the postictal period.

- Former names: Childhood occipital epilepsy of Gastaut, idiopathic or benign occipital epilepsy.
- EEG findings: Normal background associated with very frequent bilateral spikes followed by slow waves at the occipital region (occipital paroxysms; Gastaut, 1982); however, unilateral discharges may occur. Fixation-off phenomena

(epileptiform abnormality disappears with eyes open) is often present and is a valuable tool for diagnosis (Panayiotopoulos, 1981). Hyperventilation and photic stimulation do not have any impact on the recording (**Figures 9.12–9.14**).

Photosensitive Occipital Lobe Epilepsy (POLE)

- Age: Usually between 4 and 17 years old.
- Seizure type: Focal visual (simple visual hallucinations) seizures, associated with head and eye deviation as if following the visual hallucination (Specchio *et al.*, 2022). It is triggered by intermittent photic stimulation. Some patients also have myoclonic, absence and generalized tonic clonic seizures (Taylor *et al.*, 2013).
- No former names.
- EEG findings: Normal background associated with occipital, centrotemporal or generalized spike or spike-and-slow-wave discharges. These discharges are induced by eye closure, sleep and intermittent photic stimulation (**Figures 9.15–9.16**).

Self-Limited Childhood Epilepsy with Parietal Spikes and Frequent Extreme Somatosensory-Evoked Potentials

- Age: Usually between 4 and 6 years old.
- Seizure type: Versive seizures of head and body, without impairment of awareness (Demirbilek *et al.*, 2019).
- Former names: Benign childhood epilepsy with parietal spikes.
- EEG findings: Normal background, parietal spikes, and sharp waves elicited by tactile stimulation (**Figure 9.18**;

this finding is not specific of this epilepsy syndrome, and it may be present in children with self-limited epilepsy with centrotemporal spikes; De Marco & Tassinari, 1981; Fonseca & Tedrus, 2000).

Self-Limited Childhood Focal Seizures Associated with Frontal or Midline Spikes

- Age: Usually between 1 and 3 years old.
- Seizure type: Staring spell, unresponsiveness, and arm stiffening.
- Former names: Benign childhood focal seizures associated with frontal or midline spikes, benign infantile focal epilepsy with midline spikes during sleep.
- EEG findings: Normal background, small spikes in the fronto-centro-temporal regions during sleep (Demirbilek *et al.*, 2019) **Figure 9.17**.

Self-Limited Childhood Seizures with Affective Symptoms

- Age: Usually between 2 and 9 years old.
- Seizure type: Speech arrest, terror, screaming, pallor, sweating, chewing, impairment of awareness.
- Former names: Benign childhood seizures with affective symptoms.
- EEG findings: Normal background, high-amplitude frontotemporal and parietotemporal spikes, activated by sleep. Ictal onset varies, and seizures can arise from frontotemporal, centrotemporal, or parietal regions (Demirbilek *et al.*, 2019).

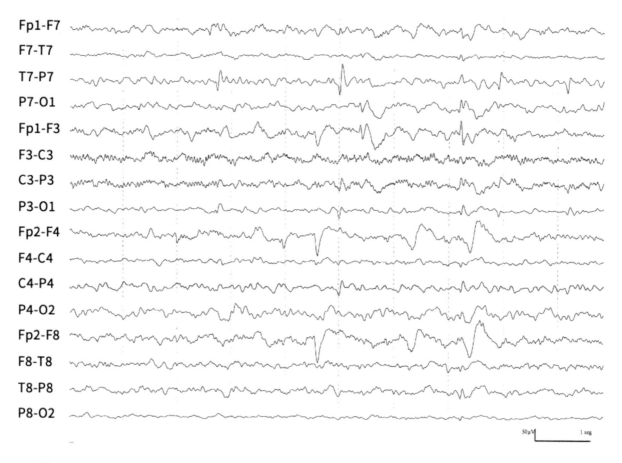

Figure 9.9 Self-limited epilepsy with autonomic seizures. EEG of a 4-year-old boy during wakefulness, showing left fronto-temporo-occipital discharges.

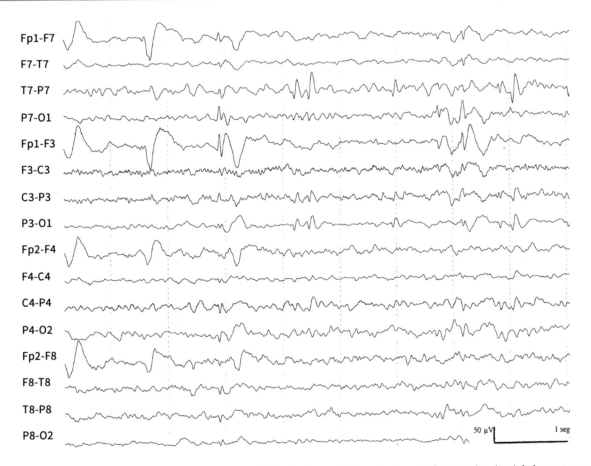

Figure 9.10 Self-limited epilepsy with autonomic seizures. EEG of a 4-year-old boy during wakefulness showing left fronto-temporo-occipital discharges with some involvement of the homologous contralateral regions.

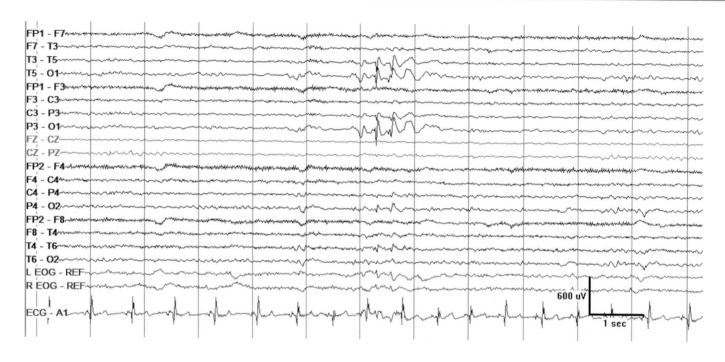

Figure 9.11 EEG of a girl with self-limited epilepsy with autonomic seizures, during wakefulness, showing high amplitude spike-wave over the left occipital region.

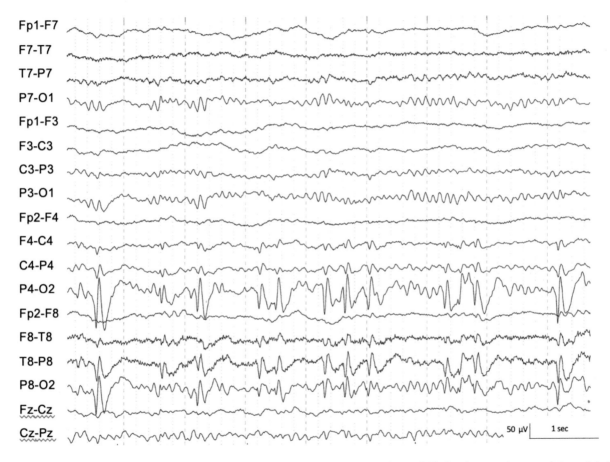

Figure 9.12   Childhood occipital visual epilepsy. Awake same patient from the previous figure, EEG showing very frequent right occipital spike and waves when the patient has his eyes closed.

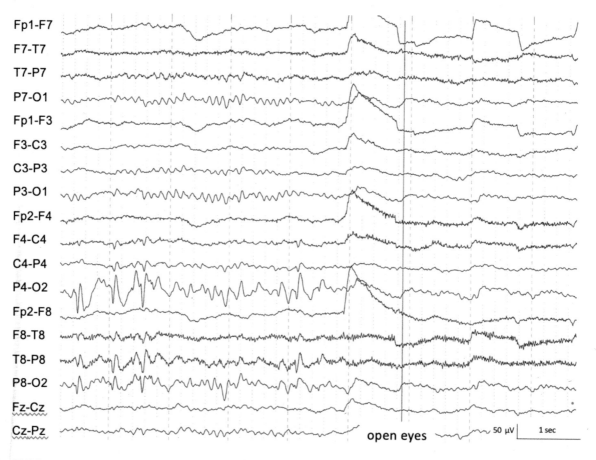

Figure 9.13   Childhood occipital visual epilepsy. Awake EEG showing very frequent right occipital spike and waves that disappear after eye-opening (fixation-off phenomena).

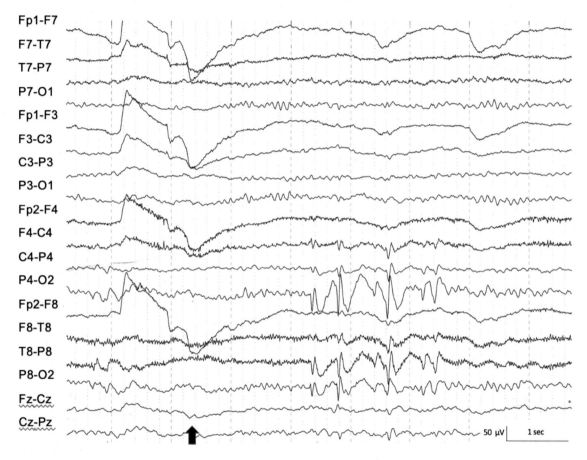

Figure 9.14   Childhood occipital visual epilepsy. Awake EEG showing very frequent right occipital spike and waves that appear 2 seconds after eye closure (arrow).

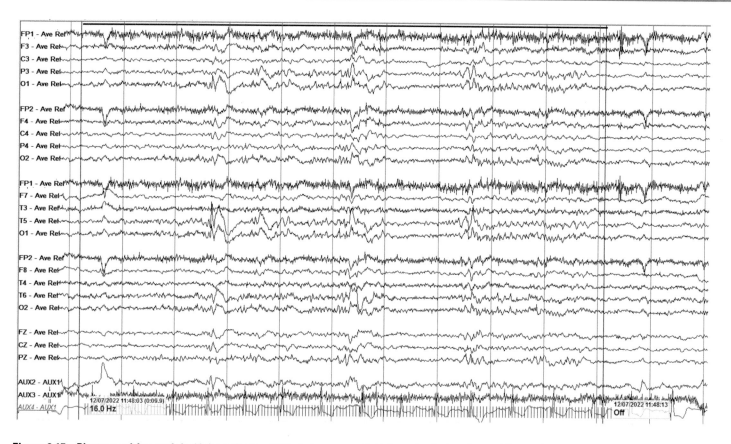

Figure 9.15   Photosensitive occipital lobe epilepsy. EEG of a teenager with history of a single seizure while watching a movie on a tablet. Intermittent photic stimulation at 16 Hz triggered spike-wave discharges over the temporo-occipital regions (left greater than right).

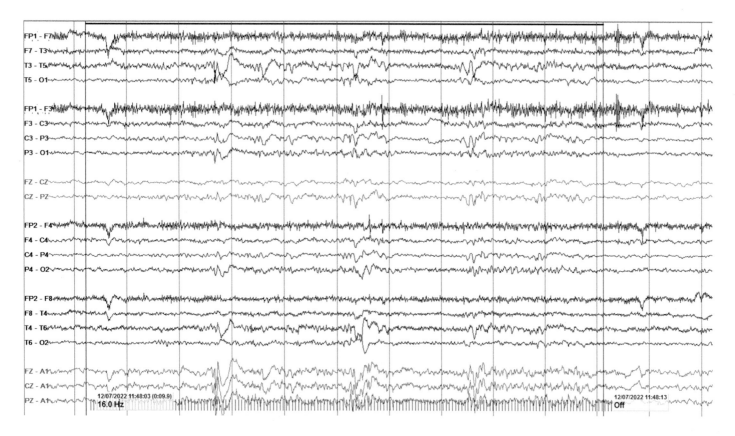

Figure 9.16   Photosensitive occipital lobe epilepsy. EEG of a teenager with history of a single seizure while watching a movie on a tablet. Intermittent photic stimulation at 16 Hz triggered spike-wave discharges over the temporo-occipital regions (left greater than right).

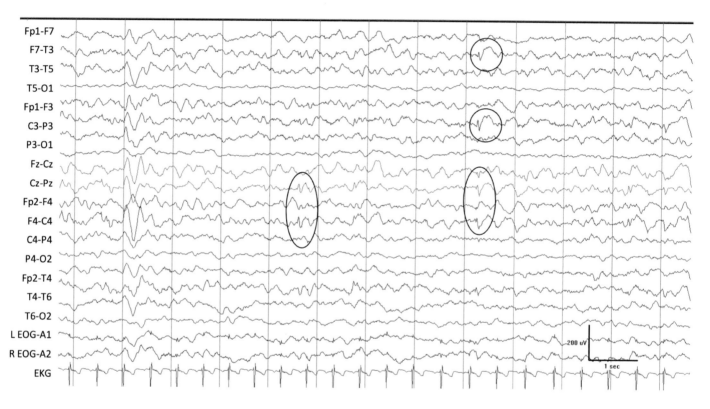

Figure 9.17 Self-limited childhood focal seizures associated with frontal or midline spikes. EEG during sleep showing low amplitude spikes followed by slow wave over the fronto-central region.

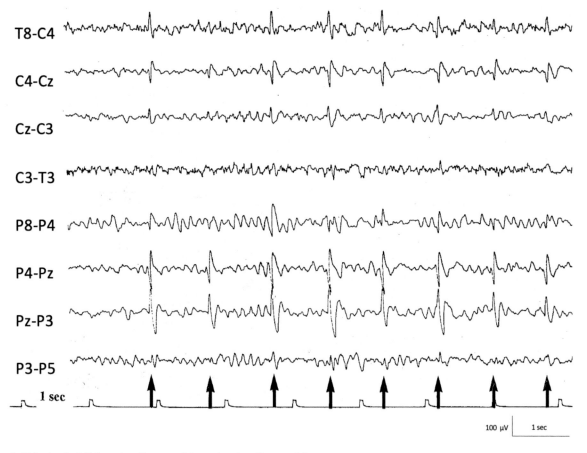

Figure 9.18   Self-limited childhood epilepsy with parietal spikes and frequent extreme somatosensory-evoked potentials. EEG showing parietal sharp waves time-locked with tactile stimulation (tapping on the patient foot).

REFERENCES

Berg AT, Berkovic SF, Brodie MJ, et al. Revised Terminology and Concepts for Organization of Seizure and Epilepsies: Report of the ILAE Commission on Classification and Terminology, 2005–2009. Epilepsia 2010;51:676–85.

De Marco P, Tassinari CA. Extreme Somatosensory Evoked Potential (ESEP): An EEG Sign Forecasting the Possible Occurrence of Seizures in Children. Epilepsia 1981;22:569–75.

Demirbilek V, Bureau M, Cokar O, Panayiotopoulos CP. Self-Limited Focal Epilepsies in Childhood. In: Bureau M, Genton P, Dravet C, Delgado-Escueta AV, Guerrini R, Tassinari CA, Thomas P, Wolf P (Eds). Epileptic Syndromes in Infancy, Childhood and Adolescence, 6th Ed. Montrouge, France: John Libbey Eurotext Ltd; 2019 p. 219–60.

Fejerman N, Caraballo R, Tenembaum SN. Evoluciones atípicas de la epilepsia parcial benigna de la infancia con espigas centrotemporales [Atypical Evolutions of Benign Partial Epilepsy of Infancy with Centro-Temporal Spikes]. Rev Neurol 2000;31:389–96.

Fonseca LC, Tedrus GM. Somatosensory Evoked Spikes and Epileptic Seizures: A Study of 385 Cases. Clin Electroencephalogr 2000;31:71–75.

Gastaut H. A New Type of Epilepsy: Benign Partial Epilepsy of Childhood with Occipital Spike-Waves. Clin Electroencephal 1982;13:13–22.

Holmes G. Benign Focal Epilepsies of Childhood. Epilepsia 1993;34(Suppl 3):49–61.

Panayiotopoulos CP. Inhibitory Effect of Central Vision on Occipital Lobe Seizures. Neurology 1981;31:1330–33.

Specchio N, Wirrell EC, Scheffer IE, et al. International League Against Epilepsy Classification and Definition of Epilepsy Syndromes with Onset in Childhood: Position Paper by the ILAE Task Force on Nosology and Definitions. Epilepsia 2022;63:1398–442.

Taylor I, Berkovic SF, Scheffer IE. Genetics of Epilepsy Syndromes in Families with Photosensitivity. Neurology 2013;80:1322–29.

CHAPTER 10

Generalized epilepsy syndromes

Shifteh Sattar, MD

Maria Augusta Montenegro, MD, PhD

Generalized epilepsy syndromes with onset during infancy, childhood, and adolescence are a heterogeneous group of genetic conditions that are characterized by generalized seizures and EEG showing generalized spike-waves discharges (Fisher *et al.*, 2017). The clinical, electroencephalographic, and prognosis of generalized epilepsy syndromes varies, with some syndromes easily controlled by antiseizure medication (childhood absence epilepsy or juvenile myoclonic epilepsy), while others are highly resistant to treatment. The seizures-types manifested by patients with genetic generalized epilepsy syndromes are:

- Generalized tonic-clonic seizure
- Tonic
- Clonic
- Myoclonic tonic-clonic
- Myoclonic-atonic
- Typical absence
- Atypical absence
- Myoclonic
- Eyelid myoclonia

Among the genetic generalized epilepsy syndromes, there are four types of epilepsy syndromes within the idiopathic generalized epilepsy syndrome (**Figure 10.1**; Hirsch *et al.*, 2022):

- Childhood absence epilepsy
- Juvenile absence epilepsy
- Juvenile myoclonic epilepsy
- Epilepsy with generalized tonic-clonic seizure alone

DOI: 10.1201/b23339-10

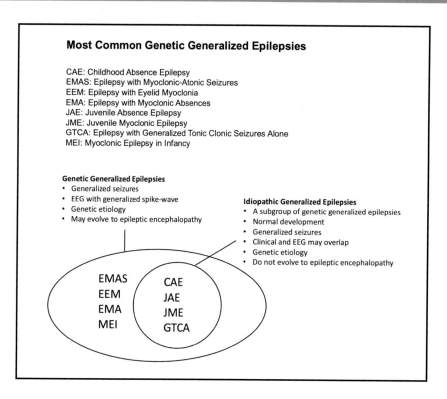

Figure 10.1   Most common genetic generalized epilepsies and idiopathic generalized epilepsy syndromes.

Patients with idiopathic generalized epilepsy have normal neurological development and can present with clinical symptoms and electroencephalographic features that overlap between the four epilepsy syndromes. The prognosis for this group is usually good, and they do not evolve to epileptic encephalopathies.

Absence seizures are seen in different types of genetic generalized epilepsy syndromes and epileptic encephalopathies. **Table 10.1** shows the different characteristics of the four subtypes of absence seizures: Typical absence, atypical absence, myoclonic absence, and absence with eyelid myoclonia (Fisher *et al.*, 2017).

In this chapter, we will discuss the EEG characteristics of the most common genetic generalized epilepsy syndromes. The genetic generalized epilepsy syndromes with a more severe phenotype will be discussed in the chapter dedicated to the developmental and epileptic encephalopathies.

1. **Myoclonic Epilepsy in Infancy**
   - Age: Usually between 1 and 3 years old.
   - Seizure type: Myoclonic seizures, involving mostly head (head drop) and upper limbs. Lower limbs may also be affected.
   - Former names: Benign myoclonic epilepsy of infancy, idiopathic myoclonic epilepsy in infancy.
   - EEG findings: Normal background with no interictal abnormalities.

Ictal findings: Myoclonic seizure: Brief generalized (anteriorly predominant) irregular high-voltage polyspikes followed by high-amplitude slow waves. The discharges last for 1 or 2 seconds, but the clinical myoclonia lasts less than a second (**Figures 10.2** and **10.3**).

2. **Childhood Absence Epilepsy**
   - Age: Onset usually between 4 and 10 years old.
   - Seizure type: Absence seizures with staring and behavioral arrest that can be accompanied with oral and/or manual automatisms such as lip smacking, blinking, or non-specific fumbling hand movements. During adolescence, a small percentage of patients will have generalized tonic-clonic seizures and develop other types of idiopathic generalized epilepsy syndrome, especially juvenile myoclonic epilepsy (Wirrell, 2016).
   - Former names: Petit mal epilepsy.
   - EEG findings: Normal background with generalized 3 Hz spike-and-wave complexes (may range from 2.5 to 4 Hz). Occipital intermittent rhythmic delta activity might also be present, usually asynchronous, triggered by hyperventilation and may correlate with more favorable prognosis (rare occurrence GTC; Guilhoto *et al.*, 2006). Absence seizures can be triggered by hyperventilation (especially if the patient has not been treated yet). Intermittent photic stimulation may trigger photoparoxysmal response in a few patients (**Figures 10.4**–**10.8**).

Table 10.1   Characteristics of the different types of absence seizures

Characteristics	Typical absence	Atypical absence	Myoclonic absence	Absence with eyelid myoclonia
Epilepsy syndrome	Childhood absence epilepsy Juvenile absence epilepsy Juvenile myoclonic epilepsy	Lennox-Gastaut syndrome Epilepsy with myoclonic atonic seizures Dravet syndrome	Myoclonic absence epilepsy	Epilepsy with eyelid myoclonia
Clinical presentation	Short duration, abrupt onset and ending	Longer duration than typical absence	Staring is accompanied by myoclonic seizures at the same frequency of epileptic discharges	Staring is accompanied by eyelid flickering
EEG background	Normal	Can be normal at epilepsy onset, but usually evolves to slow background	Usually normal	Normal
Ictal EEG	Regular spike-wave complexes (3–4 Hz at onset, but it can get slower at the end of the seizure)	Spike-wave complexes can be regular or irregular, also they can be slower (2–2.5 Hz) at seizure onset	Generalized regular polyspike wave complexes around 3 Hz	Generalized irregular spike/polyspike wave complexes around 4–6 Hz, that can be induced by eye closure or intermittent photic stimulation

Distinguishing between ictal and interictal discharges in patients with childhood absence epilepsy is controversial, but there is evidence that responsiveness is impaired regardless of the discharge duration (Browne *et al.*, 1974).

Ictal findings:

a. Absence seizures: Anteriorly predominant generalized high-amplitude regular spike-wave complexes at a frequency of 3 Hz, with return to baseline without post-ictal slowing. The complexes are not exactly at 3 Hz; they are a little bit faster in the beginning and slower at the end of the seizure. They also present a shorter amplitude toward the end of the seizure (Nordli *et al.*, 2011). Childhood absence seizures tend to be shorter and more frequent than those seen in patients with juvenile absence epilepsy.

3. **Juvenile Absence Epilepsy**

   • Age: Onset between 7 and 17 years old.
   • Seizure type: Absence and generalized tonic-clonic seizures.
   • No former names.

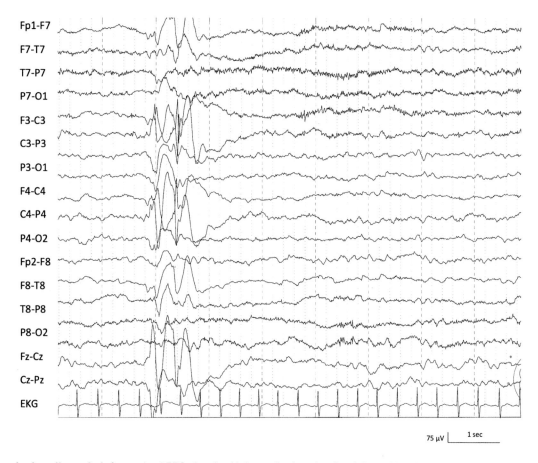

75 μV | 1 sec

Figure 10.2   Myoclonic epilepsy in infancy. Ictal EEG showing high-amplitude polyspike, followed by slow wave during a myoclonic seizure.

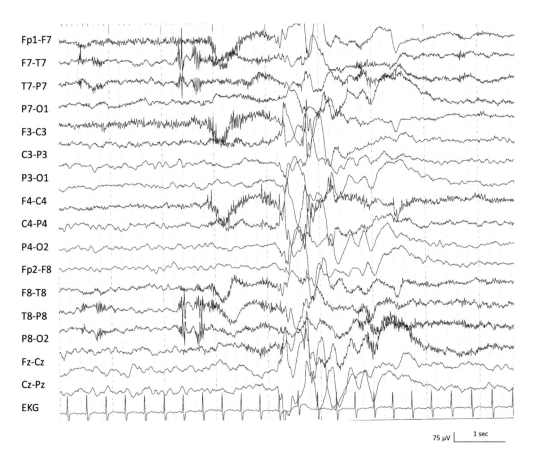

75 µV | 1 sec

Figure 10.3 Myoclonic epilepsy in infancy. Ictal EEG showing high-amplitude polyspike, followed by slow waves during a myoclonic seizure.

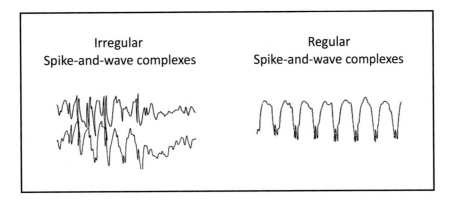

Figure 10.4 Type of spike-wave complex. Classification of spike-wave complexes according to its morphology: Irregular (different morphology) and regular (same morphology in each channel).

- EEG findings: Normal background with generalized regular spike-and-wave complexes, around 3–5 Hz frequency (the complexes are faster than the ones seen in childhood absence epilepsy). Irregular polyspike wave may also occur. Hyperventilation can trigger an absence seizure, but not as often as in childhood absence epilepsy. Intermittent photic stimulation may also trigger generalized spike-and-wave complexes. As opposed to childhood absence epilepsy, occipital intermittent rhythmic delta discharges are not present (**Figure 10.9**).

Distinguishing between ictal and interictal discharges in patients with juvenile absence epilepsy is controversial, but there is evidence that responsiveness is impaired regardless of the discharge duration (Browne *et al.*, 1974).

Ictal findings:

a. Absence seizures are like those seen in childhood absence epilepsy, but the generalized regular spike-wave complexes can be faster in frequency (3–5 Hz). Absence seizures tend to be longer, and less frequent than those seen in patients with childhood absence epilepsy, and fragmentation can occur.

b. Generalized tonic-clonic seizure: The recording can be obscured by muscle artifacts, but it is characterized by a sudden diffuse low-voltage fast activity for 1 or 2 seconds, followed by higher amplitude generalized sharp waves (around

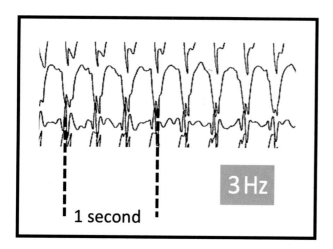

Figure 10.5   Spike and wave complex. The figure shows how to measure the frequency of spike-wave complexes.

10 Hz; tonic phase). The clonic phase is characterized by spike waves in the same frequency as the clonic movements (usually theta range). Post-ictal period shows diffuse slowing.

4. **Juvenile Myoclonic Epilepsy**

- Age: Onset usually between 8 and 20 years old.
- Seizure type: Myoclonic, absence, and generalized tonic-clonic seizures (often preceded by myoclonic seizures).
- Former names: Janz syndrome.
- EEG findings: Background is normal with generalized, irregular, 3–5.5 Hz spike-and-wave or polyspike wave

complexes. During sleep, the generalized discharges may be fragmented, but never with a consistent focal localization.

Intermittent photic stimulation can trigger generalized polyspikes wave, especially between 14 to 18 Hz frequency (Niedermeyer, 1999). Sleep deprivation may trigger generalized discharges, but the recording should be performed during wakefulness, not sleep (**Figures 10.10–10.14**).

Ictal findings:

a. Myoclonic seizures: Brief generalized (anteriorly predominant) irregular high-voltage polyspikes followed by high-amplitude slow waves. The discharges last for 1 or 2 seconds, but the clinical myoclonia lasts less than a second (**Figure 10.15**).

b. Absence seizure: Generalized regular 3 Hz spike-and-wave complexes, with return to baseline without post-ictal slowing.

c. Generalized tonic-clonic seizure: The recording can be obscured by muscle artifacts, but it is characterized by a sudden diffuse low-voltage fast activity for 1 or 2 seconds, followed by higher amplitude generalized sharp waves (around 10 Hz; tonic phase). The clonic phase is characterized by spike waves in the same frequency as the clonic movements (usually theta range). Post-ictal period shows diffuse slowing.

It is interesting to note that patients with juvenile myoclonic epilepsy have seizures early in the morning, and the same is true for the frequency of EEG abnormalities. Morning EEG recordings have a greater rate of epileptiform discharges than those performed in the afternoon (Labate *et al.*, 2007).

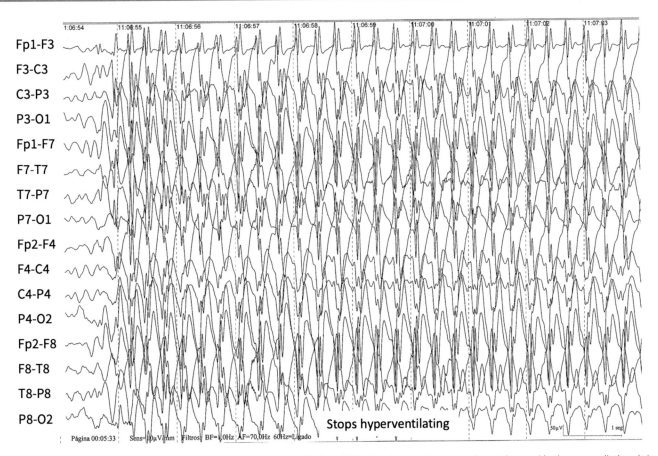

Figure 10.6   (A and B) Absence seizure triggered by hyperventilation. EEG showing an absence seizure triggered by hyperventilation. It is characterized by abrupt onset of generalized regular 3 Hz spike-wave complexes, with total duration of 17 seconds. In the third second of the seizure, the patient stopped hyperventilating and was unresponsive for the remaining 14 seconds. Note that the complexes are not exactly 3 Hz in frequency; they are a little bit faster in the beginning and slower at the end of the seizure.   *(Continued)*

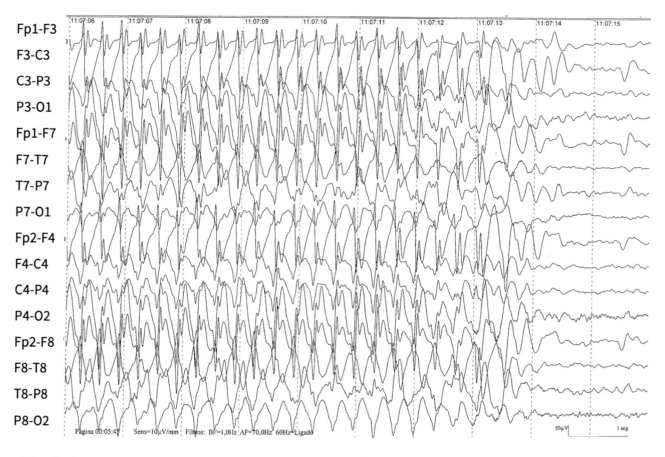

Figure 10.6   *(Continued)*

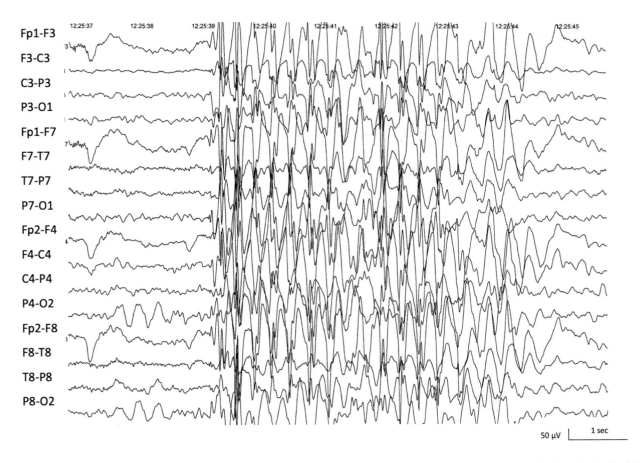

Figure 10.7 Childhood absence epilepsy. EEG showing right occipital rhythmic delta discharge (previously called intermittent rhythmic delta activity) in the first second of the recording, followed by generalized regular 3 Hz spike-wave complexes for 5 seconds.

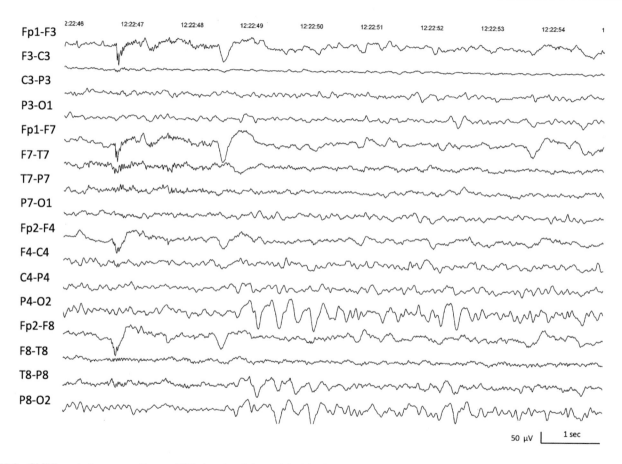

Figure 10.8   Childhood absence epilepsy. EEG showing right occipital rhythmic delta discharge (previously called intermittent rhythmic delta activity). This finding in children with childhood absence epilepsy may correlate with a more favorable outcome.

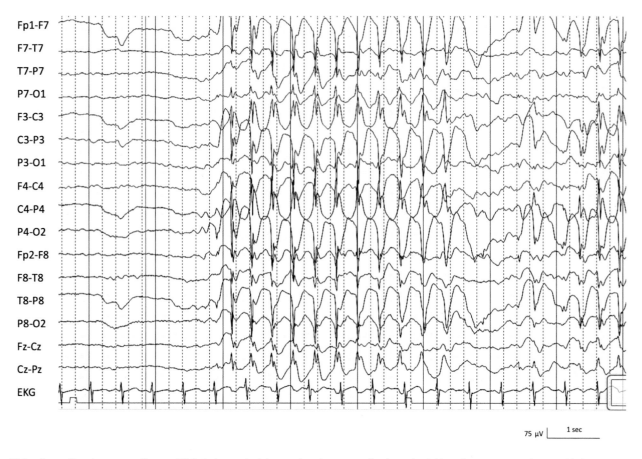

75 μV | 1 sec

Figure 10.9   Juvenile absence epilepsy. EEG during wakefulness showing generalized regular 3 Hz spike-wave complexes with fragmentation after 3–4 seconds.

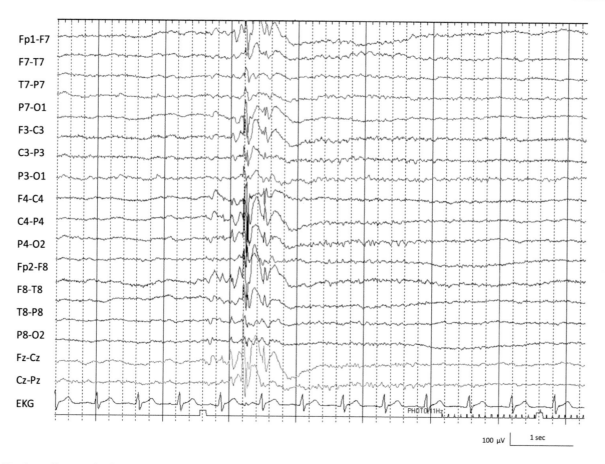

100 µV   1 sec

Figure 10.10   Juvenile myoclonic epilepsy. EEG of a patient with juvenile myoclonic epilepsy showing generalized irregular spike-wave complexes during wakefulness.

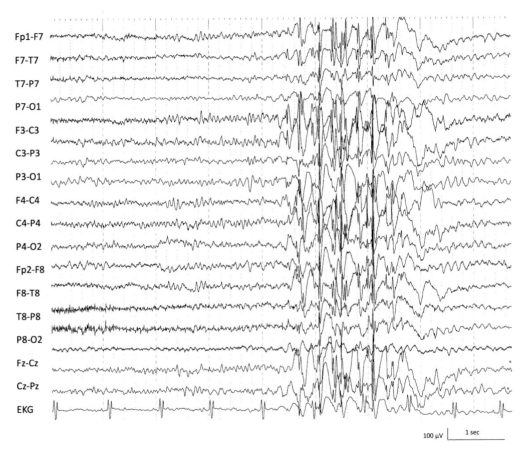

Figure 10.11   Juvenile myoclonic epilepsy. EEG of a 17-year-old boy with juvenile myoclonic epilepsy showing generalized irregular spike-wave complexes.

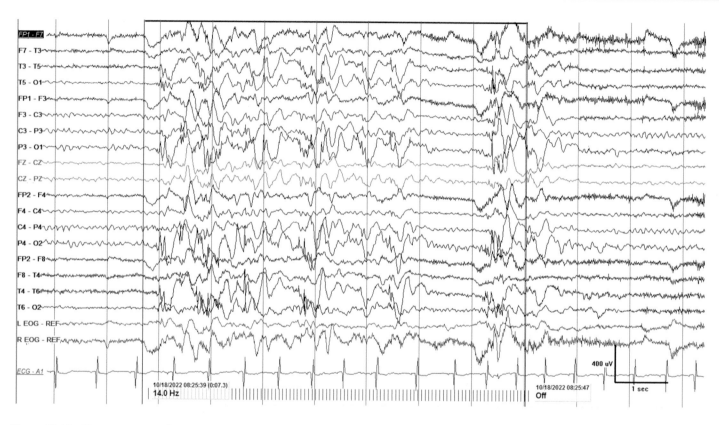

Figure 10.12 Photoparoxysmal response. EEG showing photoparoxysmal response during 14 Hz intermittent photic stimulation, characterized by generalized irregular spike-wave complexes.

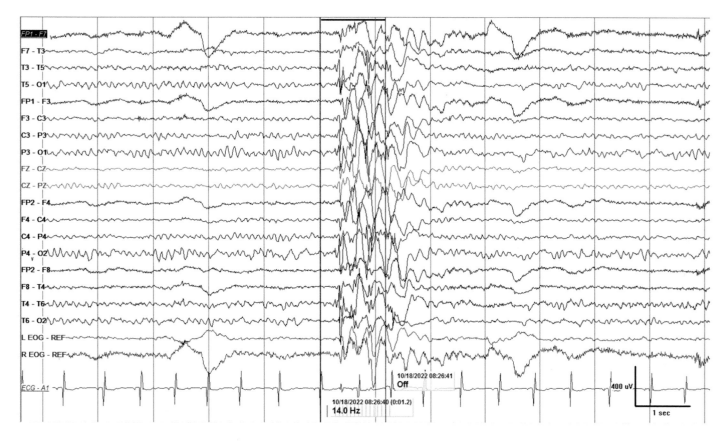

Figure 10.13   Photoparoxysmal response. EEG from the same patient showing generalized irregular spike-wave complexes when the 14 Hz photic stimulation was repeated. The photic stimulation was turned off after 1 second to prevent triggering a seizure.

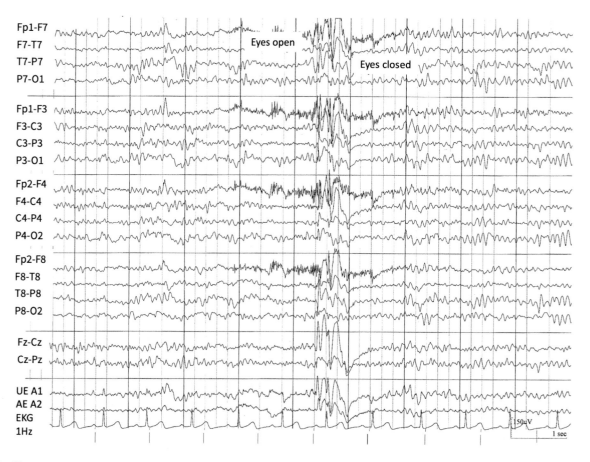

Figure 10.14   Photoparoxysmal response. EEG showing irregular generalized spike wave discharges during 1 Hz photic stimulation. Note that it was triggered by eye-opening and closure.

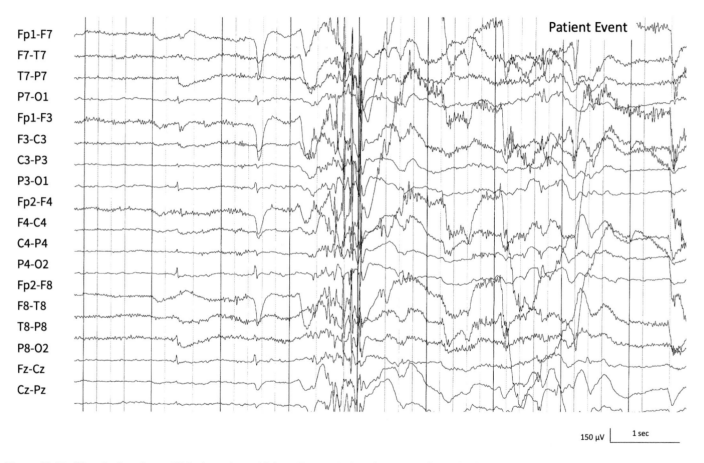

Fp1-F7
F7-T7
T7-P7
P7-O1
Fp1-F3
F3-C3
C3-P3
P3-O1
Fp2-F4
F4-C4
C4-P4
P4-O2
Fp2-F8
F8-T8
T8-P8
P8-O2
Fz-Cz
Cz-Pz

Patient Event

150 µV   1 sec

Figure 10.15   Myoclonic seizure. EEG of a patient with juvenile myoclonic epilepsy showing an ictal event (myoclonic seizure), characterized by generalized polyspike wave for half a second. During this event the patient had a myoclonic jerk.

5. **Epilepsy with Generalized Tonic-Clinic Seizures Alone**

- Age: Onset usually between 10 and 25 years old.

- Seizure type: Generalized tonic-clonic seizures.

- Former names: Grand mal seizures on awakening, generalized tonic-clonic seizure on awakening.

- EEG findings: Background is normal with generalized, irregular, 3–5.5 Hz spike-and-wave or polyspikes wave complexes. Some patients will have epileptiform discharges only during sleep. In sleep, the generalized discharges may be fragmented, but never with a consistent focal localization. Intermittent photic stimulation can trigger generalized discharges (**Figure 10.16**).

Ictal findings:

a. Generalized tonic-clonic seizure: The recording can be obscured by muscle artifacts, but it is characterized by a sudden diffuse low-voltage fast activity for 1 or 2 seconds, followed by higher amplitude generalized sharp waves (around 10Hz; tonic phase). The clonic phase is characterized by spike waves in the same frequency as the clonic movements (usually theta range). Post-ictal period shows diffuse slowing.

6. **Epilepsy with Myoclonic Absence Seizures**

- Age: Onset between 1 and 12 years old.

- Seizure type: Myoclonic absence. Absence status epilepticus and rare GTC may occur.

- Former names: None.

- EEG findings: Normal background with generalized polyspike wave around 3–5 Hz frequency. Interictal focal or multifocal discharges may occur.

Ictal findings:

a. Myoclonic absence: Generalized regular polyspike wave complexes around 3Hz frequency accompanied by myoclonic seizures at the same frequency of the discharges, followed by return fo normal background without post-ictal slowing (**Figures 10.17** and **10.18**).

b. Generalized tonic-clonic seizure: The recording can be obscured by muscle artifacts, but it is characterized by a sudden diffuse low-voltage fast activity for 1 or 2 seconds, followed by higher amplitude generalized sharp waves (around 10 Hz; tonic phase). The clonic phase is characterized by spike waves in the same frequency as the clonic movements (usually theta range). Post-ictal period shows diffuse slowing.

7. **Epilepsy with Eyelid Myoclonia**

- Age: Usually between 2 and 14 years old.

- Seizure type: Eyelid myoclonia, with or without absences, induced by eye closure and photic stimulation. Generalized tonic-clonic seizures may occur. Atonic, tonic, and myoclonic seizures have been rarely reported (seizures other than absence seizures are predictors of drug-resistant epilepsy; Smith *et al.*, 2018).

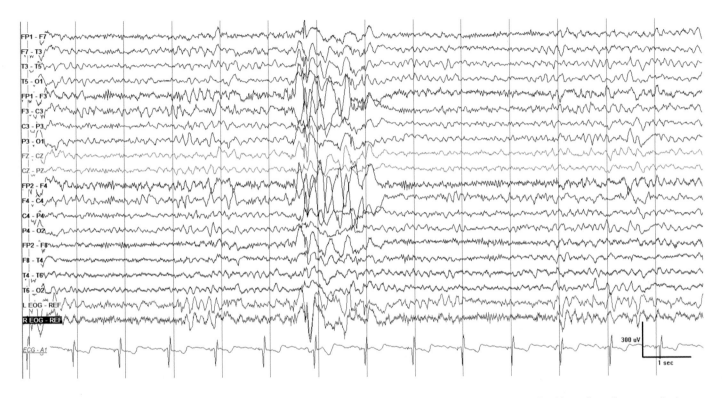

Figure 10.16 Epilepsy with generalized tonic-clonic seizure alone. EEG during drowsiness showing generalized irregular spike-wave discharge.

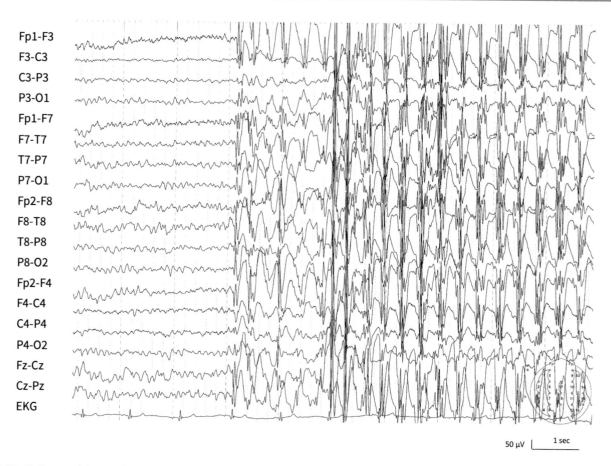

Figure 10.17   Epilepsy with myoclonic absence. EEG showing long discharge of generalized regular 3 Hz polyspike wave complexes during an absence seizure. Note that polyspikes are not usually seen in childhood absence epilepsy and when it is present, a differential diagnosis should be considered.

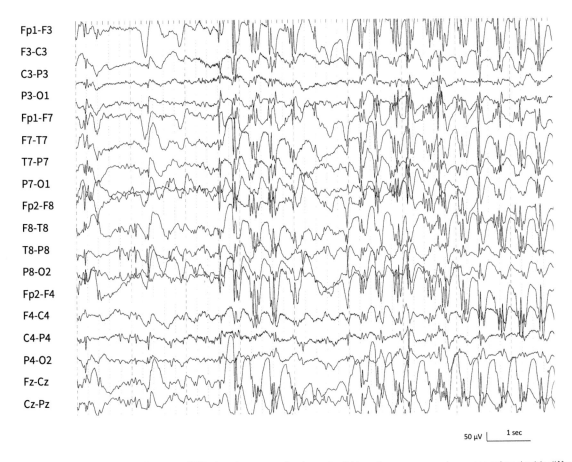

Fp1-F3
F3-C3
C3-P3
P3-O1
Fp1-F7
F7-T7
T7-P7
P7-O1
Fp2-F8
F8-T8
T8-P8
P8-O2
Fp2-F4
F4-C4
C4-P4
P4-O2
Fz-Cz
Cz-Pz

50 µV   1 sec

Figure 10.18   Epilepsy with myoclonic absence. EEG showing generalized regular 3 Hz spike-wave complexes associated with diffuse muscle arti-facts corresponding to rhythmic myoclonic seizures (head, shoulders, and arms) at the same frequency as the generalized discharges. Note that during the fragmentation of the discharges the patient did not have myoclonic seizures (no muscle artifact).

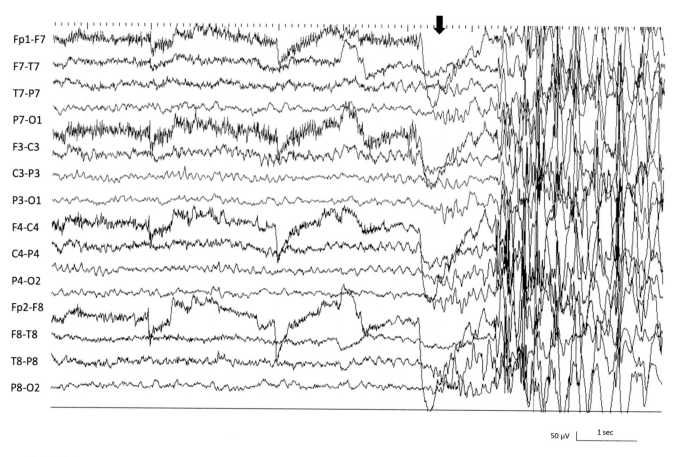

Figure 10.19 Epilepsy with eyelid myoclonia. EEG of a 12-year-old patient with epilepsy with eyelid myoclonia showing generalized, irregular polyspike-waves immediately after eye closure (arrow). Clinically, the patient presented very frequent eyelid myoclonia after closing her eyes without awareness impairment.

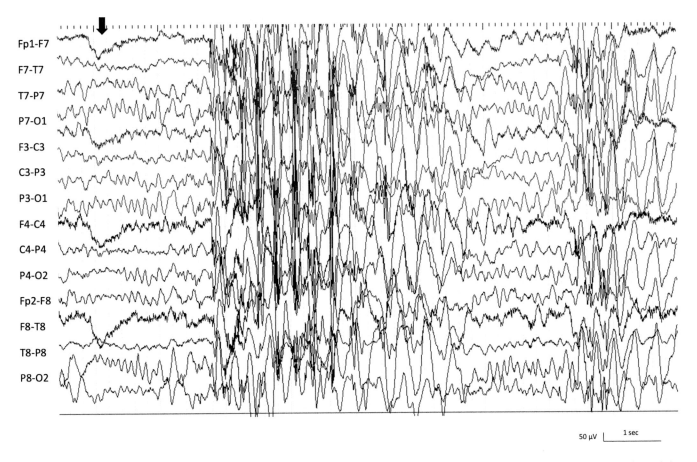

Figure 10.20   Epilepsy with eyelid myoclonia. EEG showing generalized, irregular polyspike waves immediately after eye closure (arrow). It was associated with eyelid myoclonia without awareness impairment.

- Former names: Jeavons syndrome.
- EEG findings: Normal background, generalized irregular spike-and-wave and polyspike-wave at 3–6 Hz frequency. These discharges are triggered by eye closure and attenuated by eye-opening. During sleep, the spike-and-wave discharges may be fragmented and have a multifocal distribution. Intermittent photic stimulation can trigger generalized irregular polyspikes or spike-and-wave discharges (especially in younger patients; Specchio *et al.*, 2022).

Ictal findings:

a. Eyelid myoclonia: Generalized spike/polyspike wave complexes around 3–6 Hz frequency, that can be induced by eye closure or intermittent photic stimulation (**Figures 10.19** and **10.20**).

REFERENCES

Browne TR, Penry JK, Proter RJ, Dreifuss FE. Responsiveness Before, During, and After Spike-Wave Paroxysms. Neurology 1974;24:659–65.

Fisher RS, Cross JH, French JA, et al. Operational Classification of Seizure Types by the International League Against Epilepsy: Position Paper of the ILAE Commission for Classification and Terminology. Epilepsia 2017;58:522–30.

Guilhoto LMFF, Manreza MLG, Yacubian EMT. Occipital Intermittent Rhythmic Delta Activity in Absence Epilepsy. Arq Neuropsiquiatr 2006;64:193–97.

Hirsch E, French J, Scheffer IE, et al. ILAE Definition of the Idiopathic Generalized Epilepsy Syndromes: Position Statement by the ILAE Task Force on Nosology and Definitions. Epilepsia 2022;63:1475–99.

Labate A, Ambrosio R, Gambardella A, Sturniolo M, Pucci F, Quattrone A. Usefulness of a Morning Routine EEG Recording in Patients with Juvenile Myoclonic Epilepsy. Epilepsy Res 2007;77:17–21.

Niedermeyer E. Epileptic Seizure Disorders. In: Niedermeyer E, Lopes da Silva F (eds). Electroencephalography: Basic Principles, Clinical Applications, and Related Fields, 4th Ed. Philadelphia: Lippincot Williams & Wilkins; 1999. p. 476–585.

Nordli DR Jr, Riviello JJ Jr, Niedermeyer E. Seizures and Epilepsy in Infants to Adolescentes. In: Schomer, DL, da Silva, FHL (Eds). Niedermeyer's Electroencephalography: Basic Principles, Clinical Applications, and Related Fields, 6th Ed. Philadelphia: Lippincott Williams & Wilkins; 2011. p. 479–540.

Smith KM, Youssef PE, Wirrell EC, et al. Jeavons Syndrome: Clinical Features and Response to Treatment. Pediatr Neurol 2018;86:46–51.

Specchio N, Wirrell EC, Scheffer IE, et al. International League Against Epilepsy Classification and Definition of Epilepsy Syndromes with Onset in Childhood: Position Paper by the ILAE Task Force on Nosology and Definitions. Epilepsia 2022;63:1398–1442.

Wirrell E. Infantile, Childhood, and Adolescent Epilepsies. Continuum (Minneap Minn) 2016;22(1 Epilepsy):60–93.

CHAPTER 11

Developmental and epileptic encephalopathies

Maria Augusta Montenegro, MD, PhD

Developmental and epileptic encephalopathies are defined as conditions where "the epileptic activity itself contributes to severe cognitive and behavioral impairments above and beyond what might be expected from the underlying pathology alone" (Berg *et al.*, 2010). It may occur at all ages, but it is most commonly seen in childhood. The epileptic discharges cause developmental stagnation or regression, and improvement in EEG discharges may correlate with improvement of cognition and developmental milestones. However, in some instances developmental delay is also caused by the underlying etiology itself; therefore, the term developmental and epileptic encephalopathy (Scheffer *et al.*, 2017).

Seizure manifestations are age-specific and depend on the maturation of the brain (Fisher *et al.*, 2017). During the neonatal period, EEG discharges and seizures are focal due to the lack of myelination and incomplete synaptogenesis. As the brain matures (by 4–7 months of age), the EEG shows burst-suppression, which reflects the dysfunction of thalamocortical connections. Clinically, the most common type of seizure at this age is the epileptic spasm. By 2 years old, the brain already has sufficient maturation to maintain rhythmic discharges of spikes and waves (Avanzini *et al.*, 1999), which usually correlates with multiple types of generalized seizures (tonic, myoclonic, atonic, atypical absence) seen frequently in Lennox-Gastaut syndrome and other types of epileptic encephalopathies. Therefore, the type of seizure presented by patients with developmental and epileptic encephalopathies may change as the child grows, and it correlates more with age than with the underlying etiology.

Most patients with epileptic encephalopathies have more than one type of seizure, including atypical absence seizures. Absence seizures are present in several different epilepsy syndromes, and they are classified into four subtypes: typical absence, atypical

DOI: 10.1201/b23339-11

absence, myoclonic absence, and absence with eyelid myoclonia (Fisher *et al.*, 2017). As a general rule, atypical absence seizures are associated with epileptic encephalopathies and typical absence seizures are associated with idiopathic generalized epilepsies. **Table 11.1** shows the characteristics of each type of absence seizure.

The advances in molecular genetics enabled the identification of several new mutations and have proven that developmental and epileptic encephalopathies have a much wider spectrum than previously suspected. Some developmental and epileptic encephalopathies may be caused by different genes, and also

by structural lesions, such as malformations of cortical development, vascular lesions, or hypoxic-ischemic injury. In addition, one gene may be associated with more than one phenotype, ranging from self-limited epilepsies to severe developmental and epileptic encephalopathies (such as KCNQ2 or SNC1A; Scheffer *et al.*, 2017). In this chapter, we will describe the classical electrographic features of the most common types of developmental and epileptic encephalopathies.

1. **Epilepsy of Infancy with Migrating Focal Seizures**
   - Age of seizure onset: First months of life (usually before 6 months).

Table 11.1   Characteristics of the different types of absence seizures

Characteristics	Typical absence	Atypical absence	Myoclonic absence	Absence with eyelid myoclonia
Epilepsy syndrome	Childhood absence epilepsy Juvenile absence epilepsy Juvenile myoclonic epilepsy	Lennox-Gastaut syndrome Epilepsy with myoclonic atonic seizures Dravet syndrome	Myoclonic absence epilepsy	Epilepsy with eyelid myoclonia
Clinical presentation	Short duration, abrupt onset and ending	Longer duration than typical absence	Staring is accompanied by myoclonic seizures at the same frequency of epileptic discharges	Staring is accompanied by eyelid flickering
EEG background	Normal	Can be normal at epilepsy onset, but usually evolve to slow background	Usually normal	Normal
Ictal EEG	Regular spike-wave complexes (3–4 Hz at onset, but it can get slower at the end of the seizure	Spike-wave complexes can be regular or irregular, also they can be slower (2–2.5 Hz) at seizure onset	Generalized polyspike wave complexes around 3 Hz	Generalized irregular spike/polyspike wave complexes around 4–6 Hz, that can be induced by eye closure or intermittent photic stimulation

- Seizure type: Focal seizures arising independently from multiple areas of both hemispheres (mostly from temporo-occipital regions; Kuchenbuch *et al.*, 2019).

- Former names: Malignant migrating partial seizure of infancy.

- EEG findings: Normal background at onset, but after a few weeks, background shows hemispheric asymmetry with shifting slow activity, multifocal spikes, and several focal seizures arising from different regions of both cerebral hemispheres. Seizures may overlap, with one seizure beginning before the end of the previous one (Coppola *et al.*, 1995).

Ictal findings:

a. **Focal seizures**: Rhythmic theta and alpha activity, which evolve to lower frequencies in the theta range (**Figure 11.1**), followed by spreading into adjacent areas (Coppola *et al.*, 1995). Although the EEG frequently shows several focal seizures that appear to be independent, they are actually the result of epileptic discharge propagation through the white matter fibers (Kuchenbuch *et al.*, 2019).

2. **Infantile Epileptic Spasms Syndrome**

- Age of seizure onset: Between 1 month-old and 24 months-old (most patients between 4 and 10 months-old. (most patients between 4 and 10 months-old).

- Seizure type: Epileptic spasms, often occurring in clusters.

- Former names: Infantile spasm, West syndrome. This new nomenclature includes patients with criteria for West syndrome diagnosis (developmental delay, epileptic spasms, and EEG with hypsarrhythmia) and those presenting epileptic spasms who do not fulfill all the criteria for West syndrome (Zuberi *et al.*, 2022).

- EEG findings: Although not all patients with infantile epileptic spasms syndrome will have an EEG showing hypsarrhythmia, it is the most common interictal feature of this syndrome (**Figures 11.2–11.4**). It is characterized by high-amplitude slow background associated with very frequent high-amplitude multifocal and generalized spikes or sharp waves.

Five variants have been described (Hrachovy *et al.*, 1984).

a. Increased interhemispheric synchrony, characterized by bursts of generalized spike-wave.

b. Generalized high-amplitude polyspikes and slow waves followed by sudden voltage attenuation (burst-suppression), especially during drowsiness and N2-N3 sleep stages.

c. Persistent focal spikes and sharp waves superimposed to the hypsarrhythmic background, it is usually associated with a focal central nervous system lesion.

d. High-voltage asynchronous slow waves, with only a few epileptiform discharges.

e. Asymmetrical hypsarrhytmia, persistent voltage asymmetry in a large unilateral region (or even the whole hemisphere), it is usually associated with large perinatal destructive lesions (porencephaly, leukomalacia, etc.).

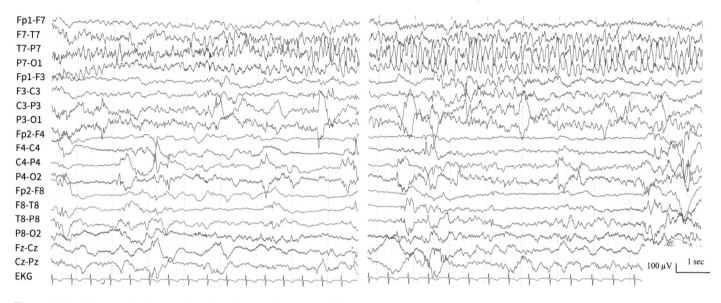

Figure 11.1 Epilepsy of infancy with migrating focal seizures. EEG of a 2-month-old baby showing a focal seizure arising in the left temporoparietal region. The seizure is characterized by low amplitude rhythmic sharp waves in the beta frequency that gradually increase its amplitude and decrease its frequency reaching theta frequency. Also note the abnormal background characterized by diffuse voltage attenuation and high-amplitude multifocal sharp waves. (Reprinted from Stafstrom & Rho, 2018, with permission).

Ictal findings:

a. **Epileptic spasm**: Sharply contoured high voltage, anteriorly predominant, generalized slow waves followed by diffuse voltage attenuation (**Figures 11.5–11.8**). Very fast low-amplitude spikes preceding or superimposed to the slow waves have also been described (Fusco & Vigevano, 1993; Kellaway *et al.*, 1979).

3. **Epilepsy with Myoclonic Atonic Seizures (Doose Syndrome)**

- Age of seizure onset: Usually between 7 months and 6 years old.

- Seizure type: Atonic, myoclonic-atonic, myoclonic, atypical absence, and generalized tonic-clonic seizures. Tonic seizures may occur but are not frequent and are associated

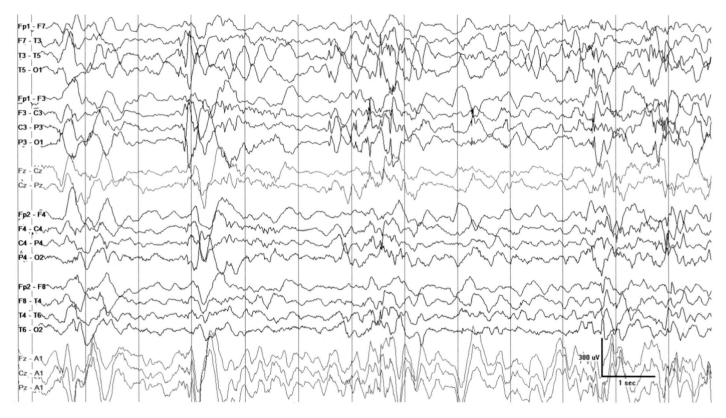

Figure 11.2   Hypsarrhythmia. Sleep EEG showing diffuse background slowing and very frequent high-amplitude multifocal sharp-slow waves and diffuse/generalized spike-slow waves, showing some degree of interhemispheric synchrony.

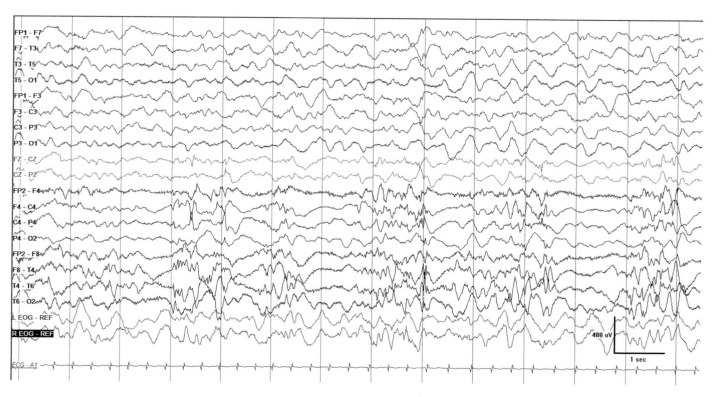

Figure 11.3   Hemi-hypsarrhythmia. EEG showing hypsarrhtymia in the right hemisphere in a girl with Aicardi syndrome (right hemisphere malformation of cortical development and agenesis of the corpus callosum).

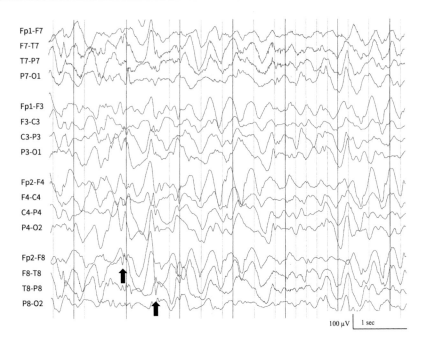

Figure 11.4   Hypsarrhythmia (slow-wave variant): EEG showing very frequent high-amplitude slow waves, with superimposed rare spikes (arrows).

with poor outcome (Kaminska *et al.*, 1999). Nonconvulsive status epilepticus is common.

- Former names: Doose syndrome, myoclonic-astatic epilepsy.
- EEG findings: Background is normal at onset, and frequently a monomorphic biparietal theta rhythm (4–7 Hz) blocked by eye-opening might be present (**Figures 11.9** and **11.10**). However, this feature is not mandatory for

diagnosis (Oguni *et al.*, 2002). With time and increased seizure frequency, there is background slowing. Interictal abnormalities are characterized by bursts of generalized 3–6 Hz spike-and-slow-wave or polyspike-and-slow wave, sometimes lasting several seconds. Some fragmentation of the generalized discharges may occur, but persistent focal discharges do not occur (**Figure 11.11**).

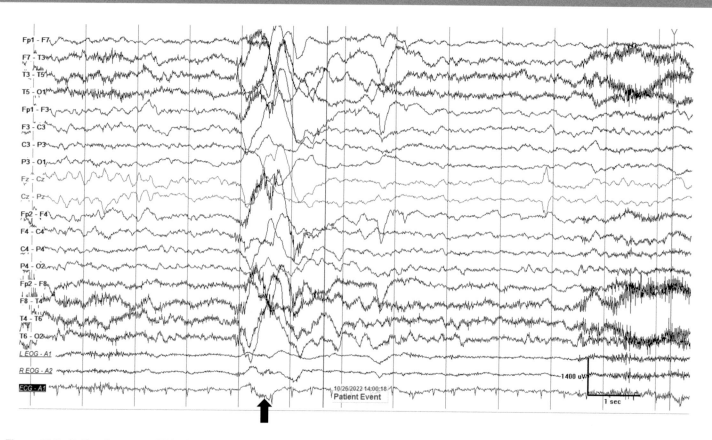

Figure 11.5   Epileptic spasm. EEG of an 18-month-old girl with infantile epileptic spasms syndrome showing an ictal epileptic spasms characterized by sharply contoured high-voltage, anteriorly predominant, generalized slow waves (arrow).

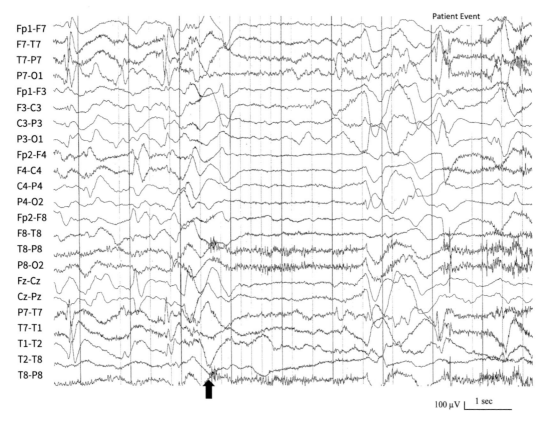

Figure 11.6   Epileptic spasm. Awake EEG showing background slowing and high-amplitude multifocal sharp-waves (first 3 seconds) and high-amplitude sharply contoured slow wave (arrow) followed by diffuse voltage attenuation for 4 seconds during an episode of epileptic spasm.

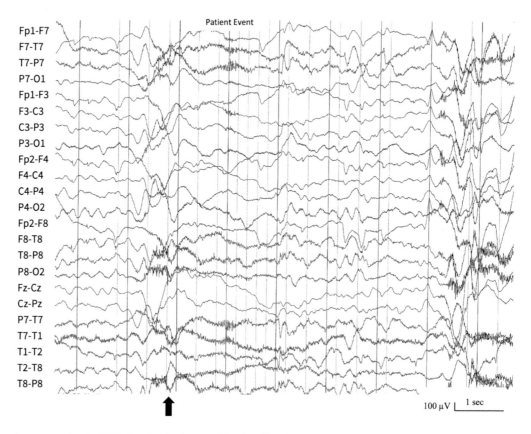

Figure 11.7 Epileptic spasm. Awake EEG showing background slowing (first 2 seconds) and high-amplitude slow waves (arrow) followed by diffuse voltage attenuation for 2 seconds during an episode of epileptic spasm. After the event, the recording shows high-amplitude slow waves (post ictal).

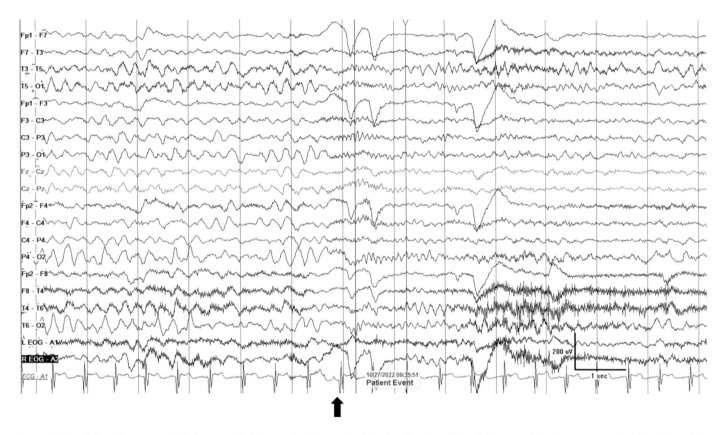

Figure 11.8   Epileptic spasm. EEG during wakefulness of a 15-month-old baby showing diffuse background slowing characterized by diffuse delta waves, followed by relative diffuse voltage attenuation associated with low-amplitude fast rhythms in the beta/gamma range that evolve to higher amplitude and slower frequency (arrow).

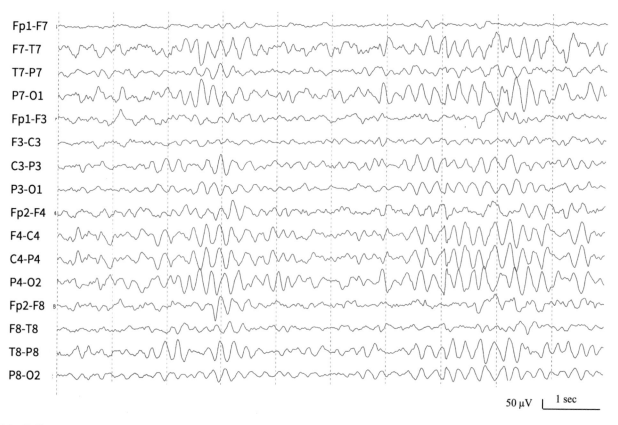

Figure 11.9   Epilepsy with myoclonic atonic seizures. Awake EEG of a 4-year-old boy with epilepsy with myoclonic atonic seizures showing diffuse background slowing and a monomorphic biparietal theta rhythm (4–7 Hz).

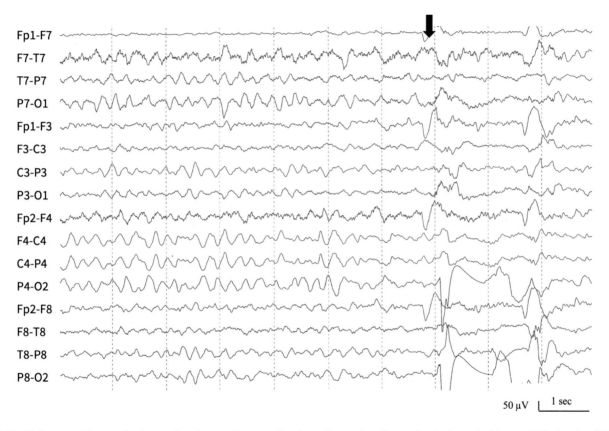

Figure 11.10   Epilepsy with myoclonic atonic seizures. Same patient from the previous figure also during wakefulness. EEG showing diffuse background slowing and a monomorphic biparietal theta rhythm (4–7 Hz) that disappears after eye-opening (arrow).

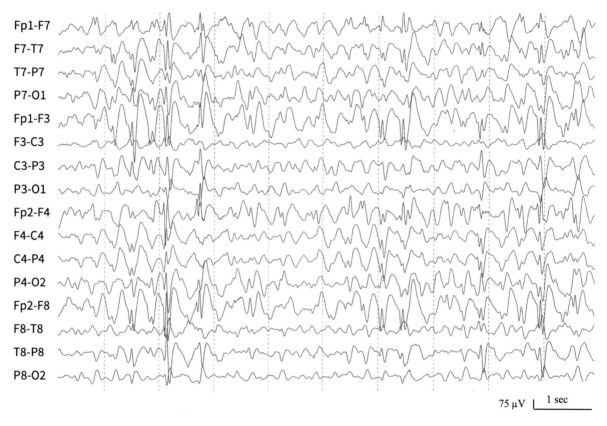

Figure 11.11 Epilepsy with myoclonic atonic seizures. Awake EEG showing diffuse background slowing and multifocal high-amplitude sharp waves followed by slow waves.

Ictal findings:

a. **Myoclonic atonic seizure**: Generalized polyspike or spike-wave (myoclonic component) followed by high-amplitude slow wave (atonic component).

b. **Atypical absence**: Anteriorly predominant spike-wave complexes at 2–3.5 Hz. As opposed to childhood absence epilepsy, the spike-wave complexes can be irregular, with variable morphology.

c. **Myoclonic seizures**: Brief generalized (anteriorly predominant) irregular high voltage polyspikes followed by high-amplitude slow waves. The discharges last for one or two seconds, but the clinical myoclonia lasts less than a second.

d. **Generalized tonic-clonic seizure**: The recording can be obscured by muscle artifacts, but it is characterized by a sudden diffuse low-voltage fast activity for 1 or 2 seconds, followed by higher amplitude generalized sharp waves (around 10 Hz; tonic phase). The clonic phase is characterized by spike waves in the same frequency as the clonic movements (usually theta range). Postictal period shows diffuse slowing.

4. **Dravet Syndrome**

   - Age of seizure onset: Usually in the first year of life.
   - Seizure type: Myoclonic, tonic (rare), atypical absence, hemiclonic, generalized clonic and generalized tonic-clonic seizures. Obtundation *status* is an unclassified event characteristic of Dravet syndrome characterized by awareness impairment of variable intensity, associated with sporadic low-amplitude segmental myoclonus, drooling, or mild increased muscle tone (Dravet *et al.*, 2019).
   - Former names: Severe myoclonic epilepsy of childhood, severe polymorphic epilepsy of infants.
   - EEG findings: Normal background in the onset of disease, but half of the patients will present background slowing as the disease progress (**Figure 11.12**). Theta waves in frontocentral regions might occur. Interictal EEG shows generalized spike-slow waves. Generalized polyspikes are seen during drowsiness and sleep (Bureau & Dalla-Bernardina, 2011). Focal or multifocal spike-slow waves might occur but without a consistent localization. Intermittent photic stimulation triggers generalized spike-and-slow waves (**Figures 11.13** and **11.14**).

Ictal findings:

a. **Myoclonic seizures**: Brief generalized (anteriorly predominant) irregular high voltage polyspikes followed by high-amplitude slow waves. The discharges last for 1 or 2 seconds, but the clinical myoclonia lasts less than a second.

b. **Atypical absence**: Generalized regular (or irregular) spike-wave complexes 2–3 Hz).

c. **Focal seizures (frequently hemiclonic)**: Rhythmic spike/sharp waves with a gradual increase in discharge amplitude and decrease in frequency.

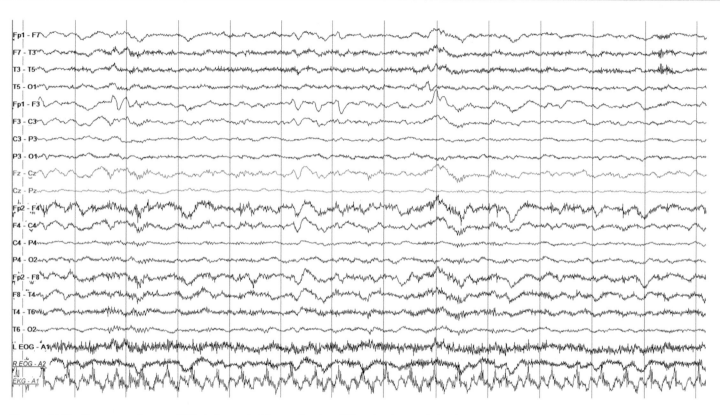

Figure 11.12   Dravet syndrome. EEG during wakefulness showing diffuse background slowing characterized by medium-amplitude diffuse theta range waves.

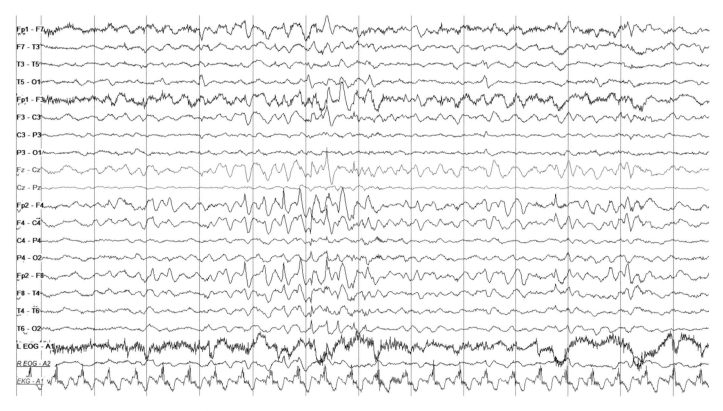

Figure 11.13 Dravet syndrome. EEG during wakefulness showing high-amplitude sharp and slow waves over the right frontocentral region, with a field over the left frontal region.

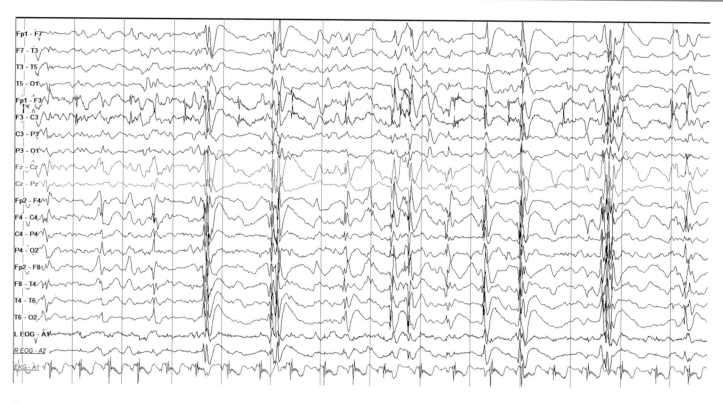

Figure 11.14   Dravet syndrome. EEG during sleep (same patient from the previous figure) showing generalized spikes and sharp and slow waves. Also focal spike and wave over the frontal regions.

d. **Generalized tonic-clonic seizure**: The recording can be obscured by muscle artifacts, but it is characterized by a sudden diffuse low-voltage fast activity for 1 or 2 seconds, followed by higher amplitude generalized sharp waves (around 10 Hz; tonic phase). The clonic phase is characterized by spike waves in the same frequency as the clonic movements (usually theta range). Postictal period shows diffuse slowing.

e. **Obtundation status** (awareness impairment associated with sporadic low-amplitude segmental myoclonus): The EEG shows diffuse slowing that might contain focal or generalized spikes or sharp waves. The myoclonic jerks are not associated with epileptic discharges (**Figures 11.15–11.17**; Dravet *et al.*, 2019).

5. **Lennox-Gastaut Syndrome**
   - Age of seizure onset: Usually between 3 and 5 years old.
   - Seizure type: Atonic, tonic, atypical absence, myoclonic, myoclonic-atonic, and focal seizures.
   - Former names: None.
   - EEG findings: Slow background associated with bursts of generalized spike-wave complexes <2.5 Hz, that are usually anteriorly predominant. During wakefulness, the slow spike-and-wave complexes may be asynchronous and focal or multifocal spike-and-waves may also be seen. During sleep, the EEG shows bursts of generalized paroxysmal fast activity (generalized sharp waves around 10 Hz) that may be associated with subtle tonic seizures (**Figures 11.18–11.21**). Intermittent photic stimulation does not change the recording.

Ictal findings:

a. **Tonic seizure**: Anteriorly predominant, high-amplitude generalized spikes/sharp waves (10–16 Hz) preceded by diffuse voltage attenuation or sharp-slow wave. Return to baseline happens after a few seconds (**Figure 11.22**).

b. **Myoclonic seizures**: Brief generalized (anteriorly predominant) irregular high voltage polyspikes followed by high-amplitude slow waves. The discharges last for 1 or 2 seconds, but the clinical myoclonia lasts less than a second.

c. **Atypical absence**: Anteriorly predominant spike-wave complexes at 2–3.5 Hz. As opposed to childhood absence epilepsy, the spike-wave complexes can be irregular, with variable morphology.

d. **Generalized tonic-clonic seizure**: The recording can be obscured by muscle artifacts, but it is characterized by a sudden diffuse low-voltage fast activity for 1 or 2 seconds, followed by higher amplitude generalized sharp waves (around 10 Hz; tonic phase). The clonic phase is characterized by spike waves in the same frequency as the clonic movements (usually theta range). Postictal period shows diffuse slowing.

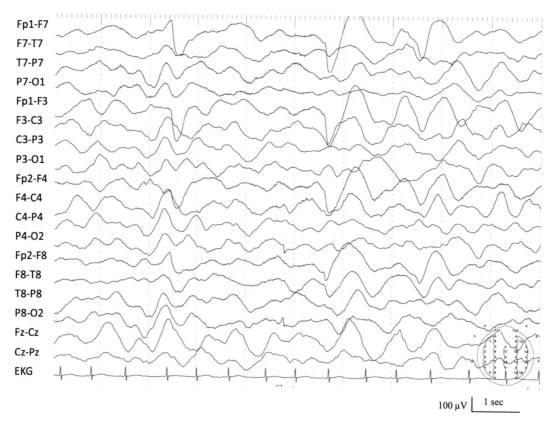

Figure 11.15 Obtundation status. EEG recorded during obtundation status in a child with Dravet syndrome. During this episode the patient was awake, but with impaired awareness. Note diffuse background slowing characterized by high-amplitude delta waves with higher amplitude in the anterior regions. (Courtesy of Ana Carolina Coan, MD, PhD)

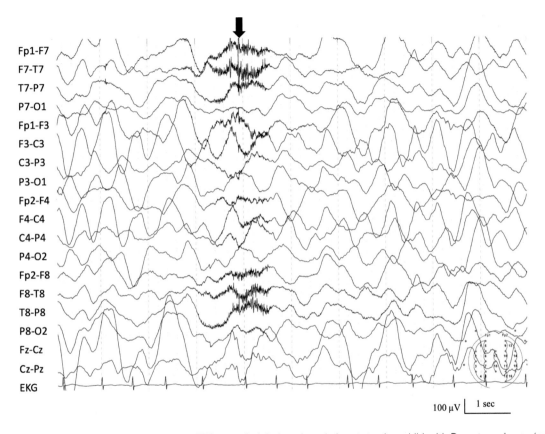

Figure 11.16 Myoclonus during obtundation status. EEG recorded during obtundation status in a child with Dravet syndrome (same patient from the previous figure). During this episode, the patient was awake, but with impaired awareness. Background is characterized by high-amplitude delta waves with higher amplitude in the anterior regions. Note that (except for muscle artifact) there is no epileptiform discharge associated with the myoclonic jerk (arrow). (Courtesy of Ana Carolina Coan, MD, PhD)

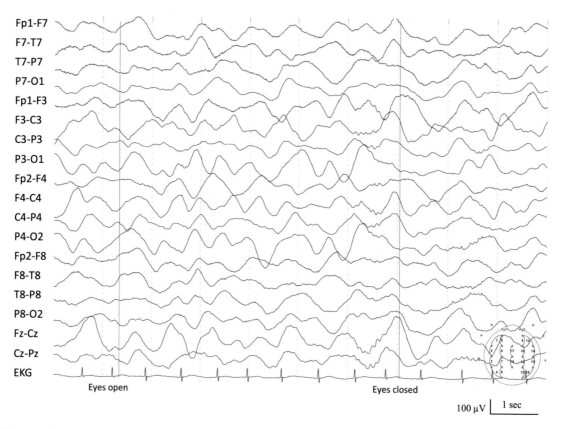

Figure 11.17 Obtundation status. EEG recorded during obtundation status in a child with Dravet syndrome (same patient from the previous figure). During this episode, the patient was awake, but with impaired awareness. Note that the diffuse slowing characterized by high-amplitude delta waves with higher amplitude in the anterior regions is not reactive to eye-opening and closure. (Courtesy of Ana Carolina Coan, MD, PhD)

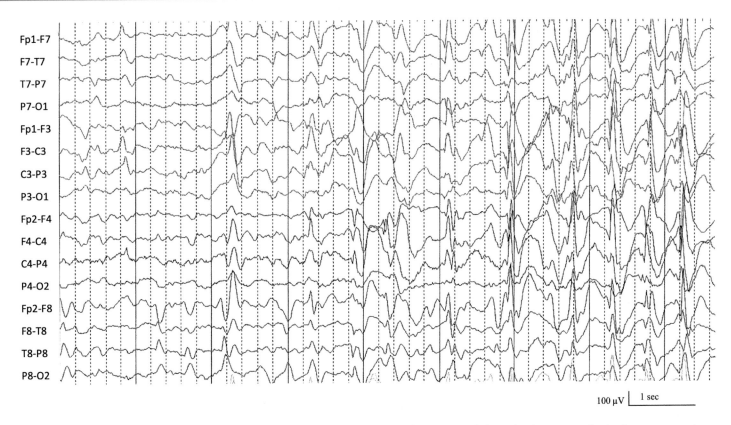

Figure 11.18   Lennox-Gastaut syndrome. EEG during wakefulness showing very frequent anteriorly predominant generalized spike-wave complexes <2.5 Hz.

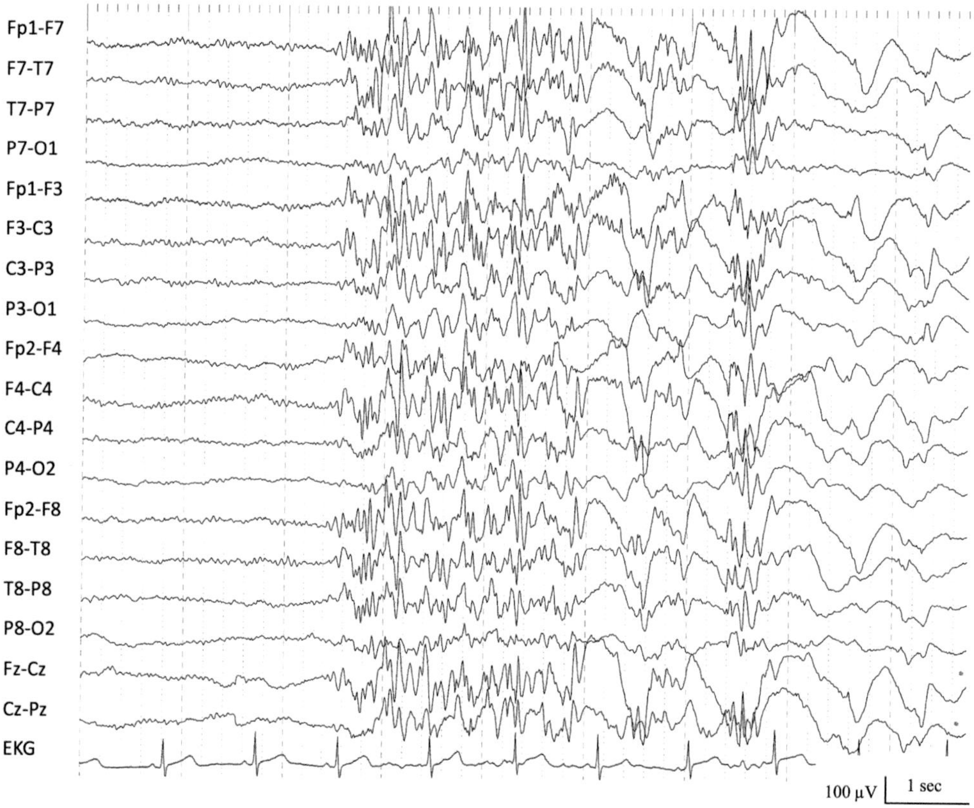

Figure 11.19   Lennox-Gastaut syndrome. Sleep EEG showing bursts of generalized paroxysmal fast activity (sharp waves around 10 Hz). This finding occurs during sleep and can be associated with subclinical tonic seizures. Note some fragmentation between the discharges.

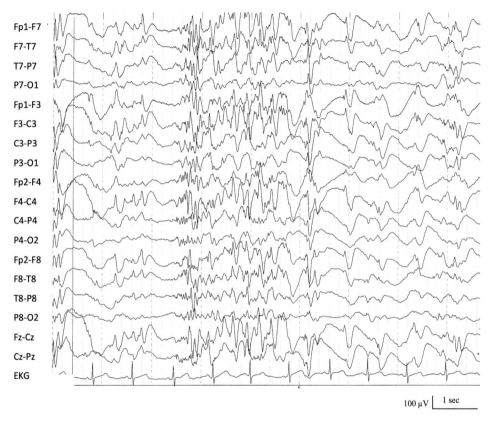

100 μV | 1 sec

Figure 11.20 Lennox-Gastaut syndrome. Sleep EEG showing bursts of generalized paroxysmal fast activity (around 10 Hz). This finding occurs during sleep and can be associated with subclinical tonic seizures.

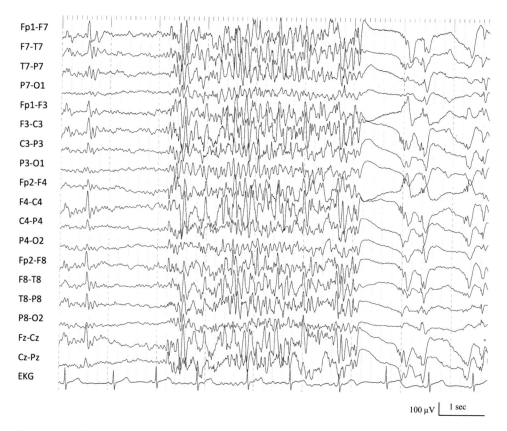

Figure 11.21   Lennox-Gastaut syndrome. Sleep EEG showing bursts of generalized paroxysmal fast activity (around 10 Hz). This finding occurs during sleep and can be associated with subclinical tonic seizures.

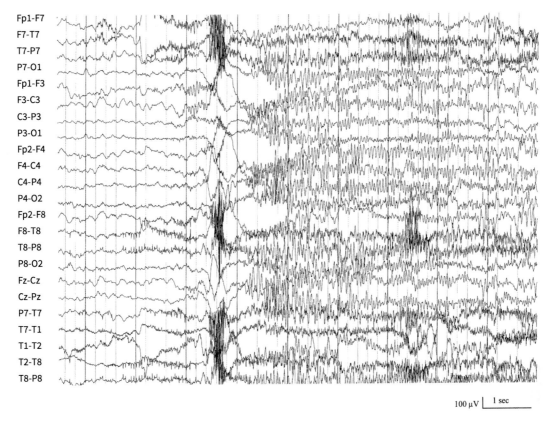

100 μV | 1 sec

Figure 11.22 Tonic seizure. EEG during wakefulness of a child with Lennox-Gastaut syndrome showing a tonic seizure characterized by sudden onset of generalized polyspikes/sharp waves for several seconds.

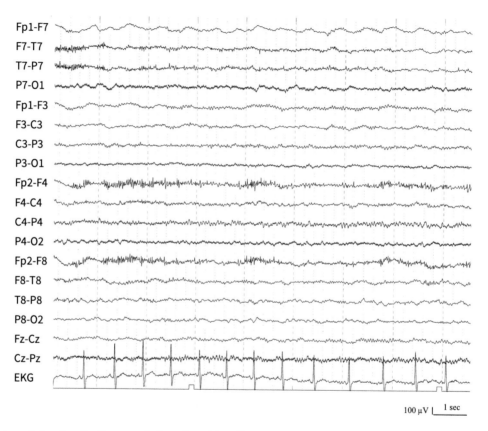

Figure 11.23 Developmental and epileptic encephalopathy with spike-wave activation in sleep. Awake EEG of a 6-year-old boy, eyes open. It is difficult to evaluate the posterior dominant rhythm, but it is clear that there are no epileptiform discharges. Note excessive beta activity due to the use of benzodiazepines.

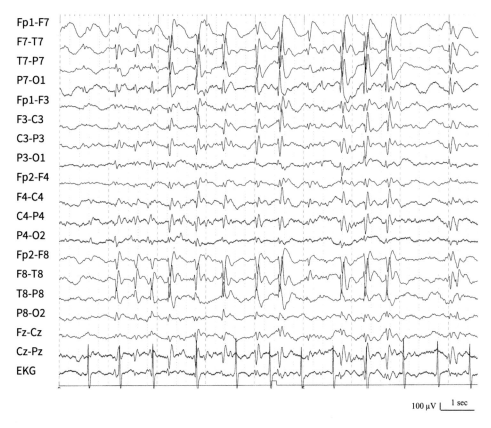

Figure 11.24 **Developmental and epileptic encephalopathy with spike-wave activation in sleep.** Sleep EEG (same patient from the previous figure) showing very frequent diffuse spike-wave discharges activated by sleep.

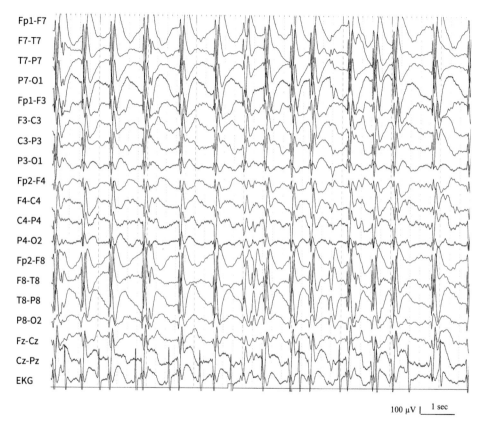

100 μV | 1 sec

Figure 11.25 Developmental and epileptic encephalopathy with spike-wave activation in sleep. Sleep EEG (same patient from the previous figure) showing very frequent diffuse spike-wave discharges activated by sleep. Note that in DEE/SWAS, there are no generalized polyspikes during sleep, which can be useful to differentiate this condition from Lennox-Gastaut syndrome if only the sleep recording is available.

6. **Developmental and Epileptic Encephalopathy with Spike-Wave Activation in Sleep (DEE/SWAS)**

- Age of seizure onset: Usually between 2 and 12 years old.

- Seizure type: Atypical absence, tonic, focal, atonic, and generalized tonic-clonic seizures. Rarely, the child will not have any clinical seizures.

- Former names: Electrographic status epilepticus of sleep, continuous spike-and-wave in sleep, Landau-Kleffner syndrome, atypical benign partial epilepsy (they are now grouped together as a single entity; Specchio *et al.*, 2022).

- EEG findings: During wakefulness, the background may be normal or show diffuse or focal slowing. Focal or multifocal spike-and-waves are frequently seen. During drowsiness and sleep, there is marked activation of the discharges, with almost continuous, slow spike-wave complexes (<2.5 Hz), often occupying >85% of N2/N3 sleep stages (**Figures 11.23–11.25**; Specchio *et al.*, 2022). The nearly continuous spike-and-wave usually disappears after adolescence.

Paroxysmal fast activity during sleep does not occur, which can be useful to differentiate DEE/SWAS from Lennox-Gastaut syndrome.

REFERENCES

Avanzini G, Sancini G, Canafoglia L, Franceschetti S. Maturation of Cortical Physiological Properties Relevant to Epileptogenesis. In: Spreafico R, Avanzini G, Andermann F (Eds.). Abnormal Cortical Development and Epilepsy. London: John-Libbey and Company; 1999, pp. 63–75.

Berg AT, Berkovic SF, Brodie MJ, et al. Revised Terminology and Concepts for Organization of Seizures and Epilepsies: Report of the ILAE Commission on Classification and Terminology, 2005-2009. Epilepsia 2010;51:676–85.

Bureau M, Dalla-Bernardina B. Electroencephalographic Characteristics of Dravet Syndrome. Epilepsia 2011;52 Suppl 2:13–23.

Coppola G, Plouin P, Chiron C, Robain O, Dulac O. Migrating Partial Seizures in Infancy: A Malignant Disorder with Developmental Arrest. Epilepsia 1995;36:1017–24.

Dravet C, Bureau M, Oguni H, Cokar O, Guerrini R. Dravet Syndrome (Previously Severe Myoclonic Epilepsy In Infancy). In: Bureau M, Genton P, Dravet C, Delgado-Escueta AV, Guerrini R, Tassinari CA, Thomas P, Wolf P (Eds.). Epileptic Syndromes in Infancy, Childhood and Adolescence, 6th Ed. Surrey: John Libbey Eurotext Ltd; 2019, pp. 139–171.

Fisher RS, Cross JH, French JA, et al. Operational classification of seizure types by the International League Against Epilepsy: Position Paper of the ILAE Commission for Classification and Terminology. Epilepsia 2017;58:522–30.

Fusco L, Vigevano F. Ictal Clinical Electroencephalographic Findings of Spasms in West Syndrome. Epilepsia 1993;34:671–8.

Hrachovy RA, Frost JD Jr, Kellaway P. Hypsarrhythmia: Variations on the Theme. Epilepsia 1984;25:317–25.

Kaminska A, Ickowicz A, Plouin P, Bru M, Dellatolas G, Dulac O. Delineation of Cryptogenic Lennox-Gastaut Syndrome and Myoclonic Astatic Epilepsy Using Multiple Correspondence Analysis. Epilepsy Res 1999;36:15–29.

Kellaway P, Hrachovy RA, Frost JD, et al. Precise Characterization and Quantification of Infantile Spasms. Ann Neurol 1979;6:214–18.

Kuchenbuch M, Benquet P, Kaminska A, et al. Quantitative Analysis and EEG Markers of KCNT1 Epilepsy of Infancy with Migrating Focal Seizures. Epilepsia 2019;60:20–32.

Oguni H, Tanaka T, Hayashi K, et al. Treatment and Long-term Prognosis of Myoclonic-Astatic Epilepsy of Early Childhood. Neuropediatrics 2002;33:122–32.

Scheffer IE, Berkovic S, Capovilla G, et al. ILAE Classification of the Epilepsies: Position Paper of the ILAE Commission for Classification and Terminology. Epilepsia 2017;58:512–21.

Specchio N, Wirrell EC, Scheffer IE, et al. International League Against Epilepsy Classification and Definition of Epilepsy Syndromes with Onset in Childhood: Position Paper by the ILAE Task Force on Nosology and Definitions. Epilepsia 2022;63:1398–442.

Stafstrom CE, Rho JM. Neurophysiology of Seizures and Epilepsy. In: Swaiman KF, Ashwal S, Ferriero DM, Schor NF, Finkel RS, Gropman AL, Pearl PL, Shevell MI (Eds.). Swaiman's Pediatric Neurology: Principles and Practice, 6th Ed. Amsterdam, Elsevier; 2018, pp. 506–18.

Zuberi SM, Wirrell E, Yozawitz E, et al. ILAE Classification and Definition of Epilepsy Syndromes with Onset in Neonates and Infants: Position Statement by the ILAE Task Force on Nosology and Definitions. Epilepsia 2022;63:1349–97.

CHAPTER 12

Ictal classification

Neggy Rismanchi, MD, PhD

Maria Augusta Montenegro, MD, PhD

Seizures are classified as focal, generalized, or as having an unknown onset. Focal seizures originate "within networks limited to one hemisphere" whereas generalized seizures start in both hemispheres at the same time. Generalized seizures are thought to be generated from deeper brain structures and then projected to bilateral cortical surfaces. Focal seizures that spread to diffusely include both hemispheres should be called focal to bilateral tonic-clonic (formerly described as a secondary generalized seizure). **Table 12.1** shows the seizure type according to the International League Against Epilepsy Classification (Berg *et al.*, 2010, Fisher *et al.*, 2017).

The electrographic characteristics of ictal events vary according to each seizure type, and their duration can range from less than a second (myoclonic seizure) to several hours (status epilepticus). When describing the ictal findings, the timing of each clinical manifestation should be included in the description. This is especially important when the clinical symptoms occur several seconds before the electrographic recording because seizure localization can be compromised.

In the neonatal period, synaptogenesis and myelination are incomplete, which precludes the occurrence of generalized seizures. Focal neonatal seizures can have the same electrographic pattern presented by older patients, characterized by rhythmic sharp waves that gradually increase in amplitude and decrease in frequency. However, sometimes neonatal seizures can begin abruptly and have a constant wave morphology throughout the whole event (Mizrahi & Hrachovy, 2016). In addition, the lack of myelination and synaptogenesis restricts the discharges to the same area, without spreading to adjacent brain regions. These features are important to be considered because the absence of

DOI: 10.1201/b23339-12

Table 12.1   Seizure type according to its classification

Focal seizures	Generalized seizures	Unknown onset
Seizures starting within networks limited to one hemisphere Focal epileptic spasm Focal tonic Focal myoclonic Focal atonic Focal clonic	Motor • Generalized tonic-clonic • Clonic • Myoclonic • Myoclonic-atonic • Myoclonic-tonic-clonic • Atonic • Tonic • Epileptic spasms Non-Motor • Absence • Atypical absence • Myoclonic absence • Absence with eyelid myoclonia	Epileptic spasm Tonic-clonic Behavior arrest

Source: Fisher *et al.,* (2017).

"build-up" and "field" in neonatal seizures should not preclude its characterization as an ictal event.

Electrographic seizures are rhythmic discharges that evolve to lower frequencies and higher amplitude and last at least 10 seconds without any clinical manifestation. The 10 seconds duration is arbitrary; however, most neurophysiologists agree that if a subclinical rhythmic discharge lasts 10 seconds (or longer), it should be classified as an electrographic seizure. In addition, the wave morphology of an electrographic seizure should be sharply contoured, but not necessarily meet the criteria for a spike or sharp wave (less than 200 ms). **Clinical** status epilepticus is traditionally described as a continuous seizure or recurrent seizures without regaining consciousness lasting greater than 30 minutes; however, in practice, most will use 5 minutes as the duration to intervene with abortive therapy. **Electrographic** status epilepticus is defined as electrographic seizures lasting more than 10 minutes or more ≥20% of 60 minutes of EEG recording (Hirsch *et al.,* 2021).

Electroclinical syndromes are characterized by entities with consistent clinical and electrographic findings that enable grouping patients in a specific clinical disorder (Berg *et al.,* 2010), which helps to guide its treatment and prognosis. Many seizures are usually associated with at least one specific electroclinical syndrome (**Table 12.2**).

Table 12.2   Most common electroclinical syndromes associated with each seizure type

Seizure type	Electroclinical syndrome
Focal seizures	Neonatal seizures Epilepsy associated with focal CNS lesions Self-limited familial infantile epilepsy Epilepsy of infancy with migrating focal seizures Self-limited epilepsy with autonomic seizures Self-limited epilepsy with centrotemporal spikes Childhood occipital visual epilepsy Photosensitive occipital lobe epilepsy Sleep-related hypermotor epilepsy Severe myoclonic epilepsy of infancy (Dravet syndrome)

(Continued)

Table 12.2 Most common electroclinical syndromes associated with each seizure type *(Continued)*

Seizure type	Electroclinical syndrome
Generalized tonic-clonic seizure	Epilepsy with generalized tonic-clonic seizures alone
	Juvenile absence epilepsy
	Juvenile myoclonic epilepsy
Absence seizure	Childhood absence epilepsy
	Juvenile absence epilepsy
	Juvenile myoclonic epilepsy
Atypical absence seizure	Lennox-Gastaut syndrome
	Severe myoclonic epilepsy of infancy (Dravet syndrome)
	Epilepsy with myoclonic-atonic seizures (Doose syndrome)
Myoclonic absence	Epilepsy with myoclonic absence
Myoclonic seizures	Myoclonic epilepsy of infancy
	Severe myoclonic epilepsy of infancy (Dravet syndrome)
	Lennox-Gastaut syndrome
	Epilepsy with myoclonic-atonic seizures (Doose syndrome)
Tonic seizure	Lennox-Gastaut syndrome
Atonic seizure	Epilepsy with myoclonic-atonic seizures (Doose syndrome)
	Lennox-Gastaut syndrome
Myoclonic atonic seizure	Epilepsy with myoclonic-atonic seizures (Doose syndrome)
Eyelid myoclonia	Epilepsy with eyelid myoclonia (Jeavons syndrome)
Epileptic spasm	Infantile epileptic spasms syndrome

CNS: central nervous system.

ELECTROGRAPHIC AND CLINICAL CHARACTERISTICS OF EACH SEIZURE TYPE

Focal seizure

Clinical characteristics: Seizure presentation depends on the cortical localization of seizure onset (Chowdhury *et al.*, 2021; **Table 12.3**). Focal impaired awareness seizures are focal seizures that have extended to impair patient responsiveness and can appear similar to an absence seizure but typically are longer, have a post-ictal phase, and sometimes can be preceded by an aura or warning that the seizure is starting (again depending on seizure onset zone). Some may simply stop and stare during this seizure, but many can present with automatisms such as lip smacking, clothes picking, walking aimlessly, or repeating a phrase.

Electrographic characteristics: It starts with fast frequency rhythmic spikes/sharp waves, or spike/sharp-slow waves that evolve to a slower frequency and higher amplitude. It also spreads to adjacent or homologous contralateral regions (**Figures 12.1 and 12.2**). It may evolve to a bilateral tonic-clonic seizure (formerly called secondary generalized seizure).

Generalized tonic-clonic seizure

Clinical characteristics: Bilateral and symmetrical tonic posturing, characterized by arms extension in supination, followed by bilateral clonic jerking that slows over time until the seizure stops.

Electrographic characteristics: EEG can be obscured by muscle artifact, but it is characterized by a sudden diffuse decrease in

Table 12.3   Most common localizing symptoms

Seizure symptom	Localization
Figure of four sign	Extended arm is contralateral to seizure onset in frontal lobe.
Hyperkinetic symptoms	Frontal lobe. It is not a lateralizing symptom.
Clonic movements	Contralateral frontal lobe (primary motor cortex).
Fencing posture	Extended arm is contralateral to seizure onset in mesial frontal lobe (supplementary motor area).
Chapeau de gendarme	Frontal lobe (anterior cingulate, orbitofrontal region, mesio-prefrontal or premotor cortex). It is not a lateralizing symptom.
Asymmetric clonic ending after focal to bilateral tonic-clonic seizure	Last clonic jerk is ipsilateral to seizure onset.
Rising epigastric sensation, abdominal discomfort	Mesial temporal lobe. It is not a lateralizing symptom.
Déjà vu	Mesial temporal lobe. It is not a lateralizing symptom.
Dystonic hand posture	Contralateral hippocampus.
Nose wiping (post-ictal)	Ipsilateral hippocampus.
Gustatory symptom	Peri-Rolandic, insular, and opercular regions. It is not a lateralizing symptom.
Olfactory symptom	Amygdala, piriform cortex and uncus, orbitofrontal cortex, insula. It is not a lateralizing symptom.
Fear	Amygdala. It is not a lateralizing symptom.
Laughter (gelastic seizure)	Hypothalamus (hypothalamic hamartoma). Also, cingulate gyrus, frontal and temporal lobe. This is not a lateralizing symptom.
Somatosensory (pain, tingling, paresthesia): Parietal lobe	Contralateral parietal lobe.
Visual symptoms (usually elementary)	Occipital lobe. This is not a lateralizing symptom.
Nystagmus	Occipital lobe (fast phase is most often contralateral to seizure onset).
Elaborate auditory features (voices, music, etc.)	Auditory association area, superior temporal gyrus. It is not a lateralizing symptom.
Elementary auditory symptoms (humming, ringing, buzzing, etc.)	Primary auditory cortex (Heschl's gyrus in the temporal lobe). If unilateral, may be contralateral to seizure onset.

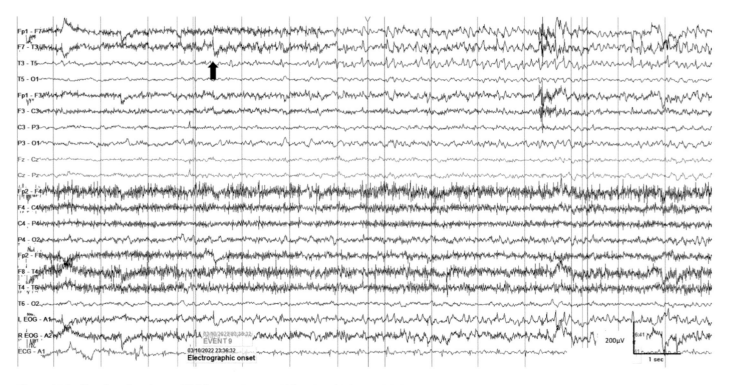

Figure 12.1 Focal tonic seizure. EEG from a 16-year-old female with intractable focal epilepsy showing an irregular left temporal (F7, T3) sharp wave pattern (starting at black arrow), which evolves to be more regular and increased in amplitude and decreases in frequency over time. Clinically, patient was noted to have behavioral arrest with this event.

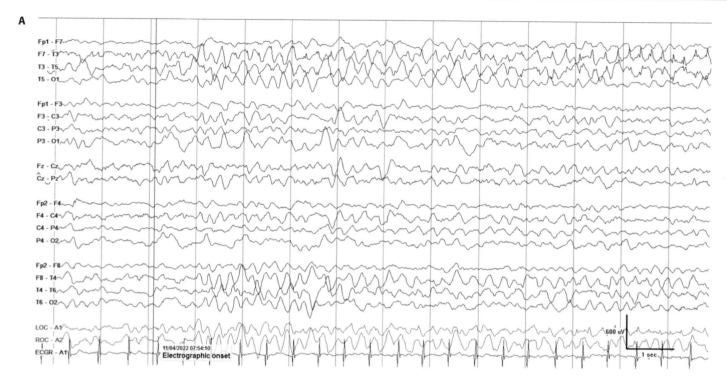

Figure 12.2   (A) Focal seizure onset. EEG showing rhythmic left temporal sharply contoured theta wave pattern, which evolves to spike-wave morphology with progressive increase in amplitude and decrease in frequency over time. **(B) Seizure evolution. (C) Seizure offset.**   *(Continued)*

B

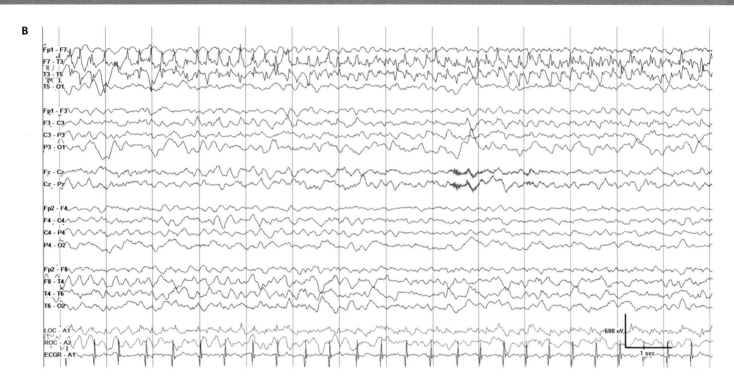

Figure 12.2   *(Continued)*

C

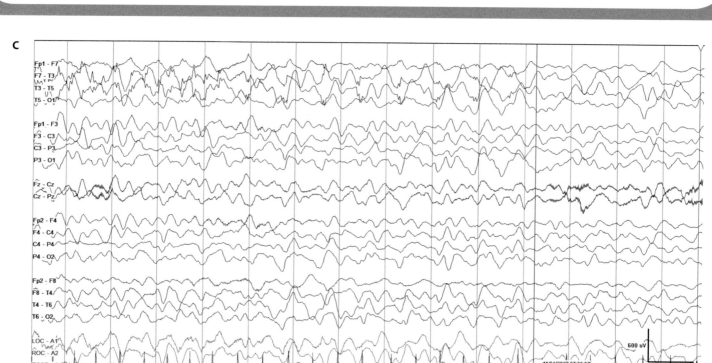

Figure 12.2   *(Continued)*

voltage for 1 or 2 seconds, followed by generalized fast frequency (around 10 Hz) sharp waves that lasts several seconds (tonic phase). The clonic phase is characterized by generalized spike waves in the same frequency as the clonic movements (usually theta range), which typically slows over time to a delta-range frequency. The post-ictal period appears as diffuse slowing (**Figure 12.3**).

Absence seizure

Clinical characteristics: Sudden onset characterized by blank out or staring spells for about 5–20 seconds. During the seizure, the patient may have eyelid flutter, lip-smacking, chewing movements, or automatic hand movements. It ends abruptly, without post-ictal symptoms.

Electrographic characteristics: Anteriorly predominant, generalized, high-amplitude, regular, spike-wave complexes at a frequency of 3 Hz, with a return to baseline typically with an abrupt onset and offset. The complexes are not exactly at 3 Hz; they are a little bit faster in the beginning (closer to 3.5–4 Hz) and slower at the end of the seizure (**Figure 12.4**). They also present a shorter amplitude toward the end of the seizure (Nordli *et al.*, 2011). Childhood absence seizures tend to be shorter and more frequent than those seen in patients with juvenile absence epilepsy. The spike-wave complexes in patients with juvenile absence epilepsy can be faster (3–5 Hz) than the ones seen in childhood absence epilepsy.

Atypical absence seizure

Clinical characteristics: Generally, these seizures have a more gradual onset and offset than what is noted in typical absence

seizures, with staring spells for about 10–30 seconds. During the seizure, the patient may have eyelid flutter, lip-smacking, chewing movements, or automatic hand movements. It ends abruptly, without post-ictal symptoms. These seizures can also be associated with loss of muscle tone of the head or trunk as well as subtle myoclonic jerks.

Electrographic characteristics: Anteriorly predominant spike-wave complexes at 2–3.5 Hz. As opposed to childhood absence epilepsy, the spike-wave complexes can be irregular, with variable morphology (**Figure 12.5**).

Myoclonic absence

Clinical characteristics: Sudden onset of staring spell for about 5–20 seconds accompanied by rhythmic jerks of the upper limbs (usually bilateral and symmetric but can be asymmetric) that occur at the same frequency and are time-locked to the 3–3.5 Hz spike and wave on the EEG.

Electrographic characteristics: Anteriorly predominant, generalized, high-amplitude regular spike-wave complexes at a frequency of 3 Hz, with return to baseline without post-ictal slowing. EMG channels show fast muscle activity (myoclonias) at the same frequency as the epileptic discharges (**Figure 12.6**).

Myoclonic seizure

Clinical characteristics: Sudden jerk that lasts less than 1 second and is usually bilateral and symmetric but can be asymmetric. It may occur in clusters and are less organized than the rhythmic jerking of clonic seizures.

A

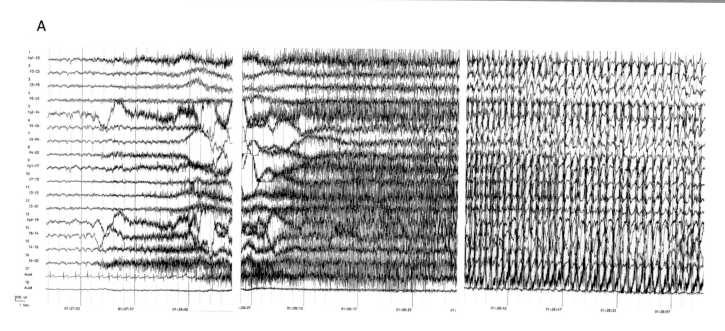

Figure 12.3   (A) Generalized tonic-clonic seizure. EEG showing sudden diffuse decrease in voltage, followed by generalized fast frequency (around 10 Hz) polyspikes that last several seconds (tonic phase). The clonic phase (3rd panel) is characterized by generalized spike waves in the same frequency as the clonic movements (usually theta range), which typically slows over time to a delta-range frequency. The post-ictal period appears as diffuse slowing. **(B) Generalized tonic clonic seizure (continued).** EEG showing that the frequency of the generalized spike waves slows over time to a delta-range frequency (1st panel). The post-ictal period appears as diffuse slowing (2nd and 3rd panels).   *(Continued)*

B

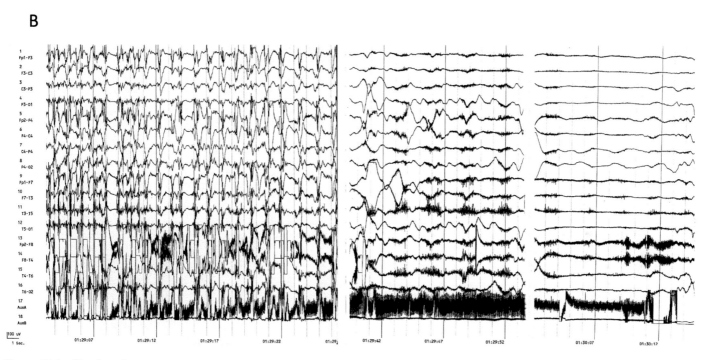

Figure 12.3 *(Continued)*

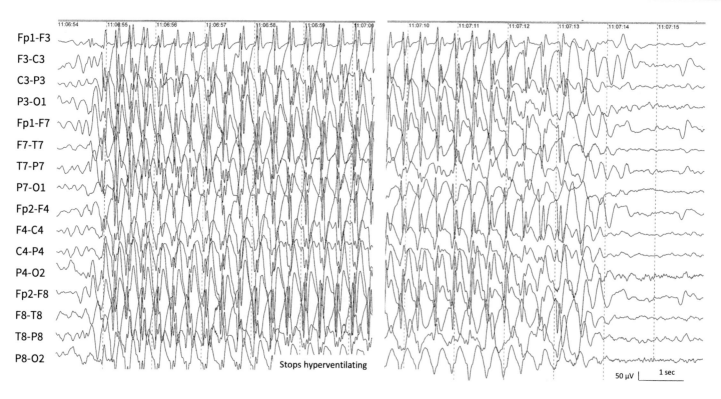

Figure 12.4　Typical absence. EEG showing an absence seizure triggered by hyperventilation. It is characterized by the abrupt onset of generalized regular 3 Hz spike-wave complexes, with a total duration of 17 seconds.

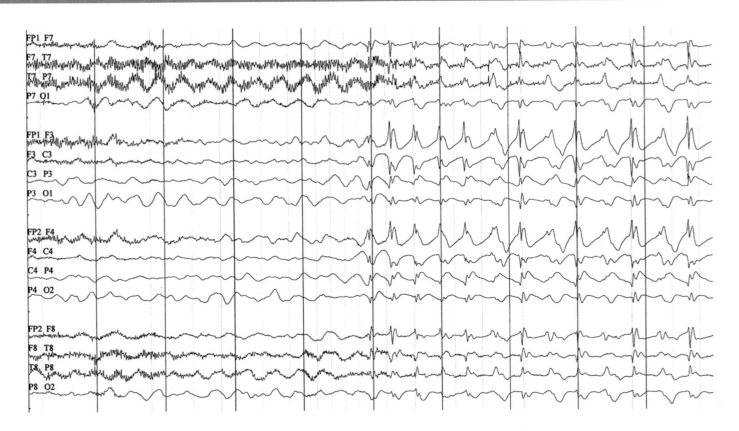

Figure 12.5 Atypical absence seizure. EEG showing diffuse background slowing and sudden onset of generalized 2.5–3 Hz spike-wave complex.

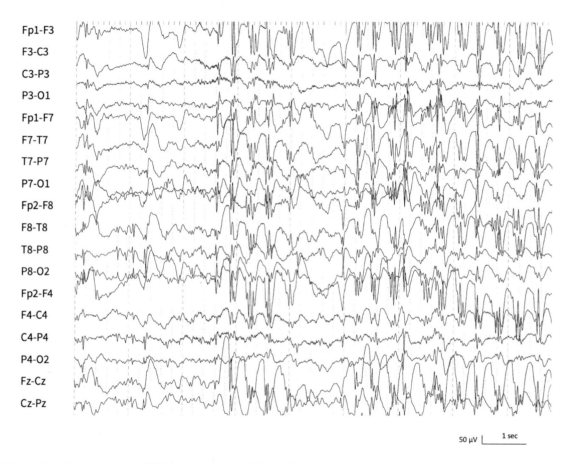

50 µV | 1 sec

Figure 12.6 Myoclonic absence seizure. EEG from a 15-year-old boy with epilepsy with myoclonic absence showing generalized 3 Hz polyspike-wave complexes during a myoclonic absence seizure. Note that polyspikes are not usually seen in childhood absence epilepsy and, when it is present, a differential diagnosis should be considered.

Electrographic characteristics: Brief generalized (anteriorly predominant) irregular high-voltage polyspikes followed by high-amplitude slow waves. The discharges last for 1 or 2 seconds (especially the slow wave component), but the clinical myoclonia lasts less than a second (**Figures 12.7** and **12.8**).

Myoclonic atonic seizure

Clinical characteristics: Sudden jerks of the upper extremities followed by loss of muscle tone, which causes head drop or a whole-body fall if standing.

Electrographic characteristics: Generalized polyspike or spike-wave (myoclonic component) followed by high-amplitude slow wave (atonic component; **Figure 12.9**).

Atonic seizures

Clinical characteristics: Sudden loss of muscle tone that may affect the whole body (causing the patient to fall) or only one group of muscles causing head drop or limb atonia.

Electrographic characteristics: Generalized high-amplitude spike or polyspike-wave discharge.

Tonic seizure

Clinical characteristics: Sudden muscular contraction, usually affecting extensor muscles, however, it may also affect flexor muscles. It can be focal (affecting only one limb) or generalized (affecting arms, legs, and truncal muscles in a symmetric or asymmetric way). Tonic seizures are frequently associated with epileptic encephalopathies.

Electrographic characteristics: Anteriorly predominant, high-amplitude generalized spikes/sharp waves (10–16 Hz) preceded by diffuse voltage attenuation or sharp-slow wave (**Figure 12.10**). Return to baseline happens after a few seconds.

Epileptic spasm

Clinical characteristics: Sudden flexion or extension of axial muscles including head, arms, and legs, with sustained tonic posturing lasting 0.5 to 2 seconds. Upward eye deviation is frequently seen. They usually occur in clusters with intervals of several seconds between each epileptic spasm.

Electrographic characteristics: Sharply contoured high-voltage, anteriorly predominant, generalized slow waves followed by diffuse voltage attenuation. Very fast low-amplitude spikes preceding or superimposed to the slow waves have also been described (**Figures 12.11** and **12.12**; Fusco & Vigevano, 1993, Kellaway *et al.*, 1979).

Eyelid myoclonia

Clinical characteristics: Eye flickering movements triggered by eye closure that may or may not be accompanied by awareness impairment/absence seizure.

Electrographic characteristics: Generalized irregular spike/polyspike wave complexes around 3–6 Hz, that can be induced by eye closure (**Figure 12.13**) or intermittent photic stimulation.

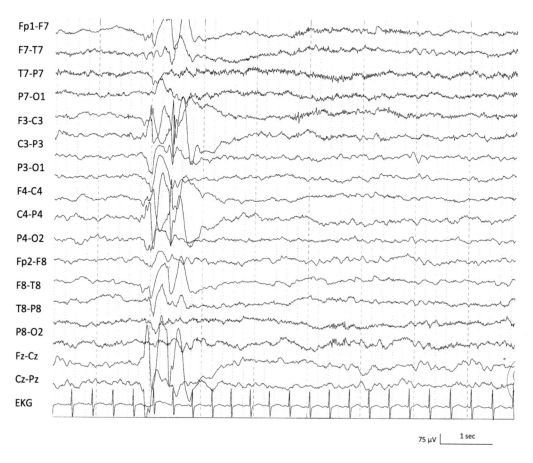

75 µV | 1 sec

Figure 12.7 Myoclonic seizure. EEG from a child with myoclonic epilepsy of infancy showing high-amplitude polyspike-wave, followed by slow waves during a myoclonic seizure.

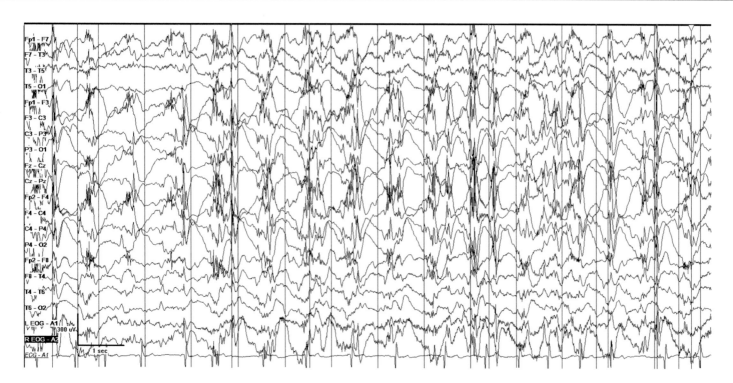

Figure 12.8   Myoclonic seizure. This EEG is from a 7-year-old male with epilepsy who had a series of whole-body brief jerks that lasted for 20 seconds. The EEG demonstrates a series of irregular, high-amplitude polyspikes followed by high-amplitude slow waves, most of which were associated with myoclonic jerks.

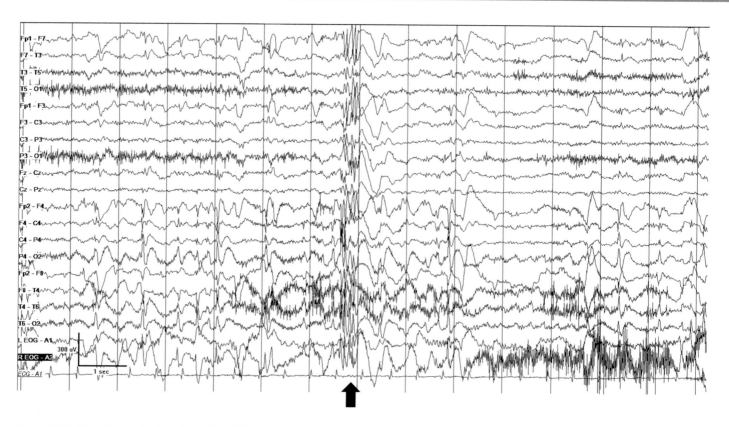

Figure 12.9   Myoclonic atonic seizure. This EEG is from an 11-year-old male with epilepsy who was having clinical spells of brief loss of truncal tone preceded by subtle myoclonic jerk. The EEG demonstrates a generalized polyspike followed by high-amplitude slow wave (denoted by the arrow), at which time patient was seen to have a whole-body twitch and fell to his side.

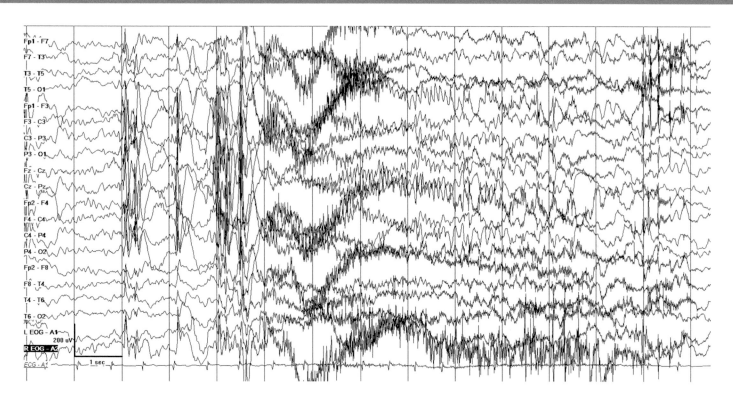

Figure 12.10   Tonic seizure. This EEG is from a 7-year-old male with intractable generalized epilepsy. The EEG demonstrates generalized fast (10–16 Hz) activity preceded by diffuse polyspike-slow wave. Note there is movement artifact at the onset of the tonic stiffening.

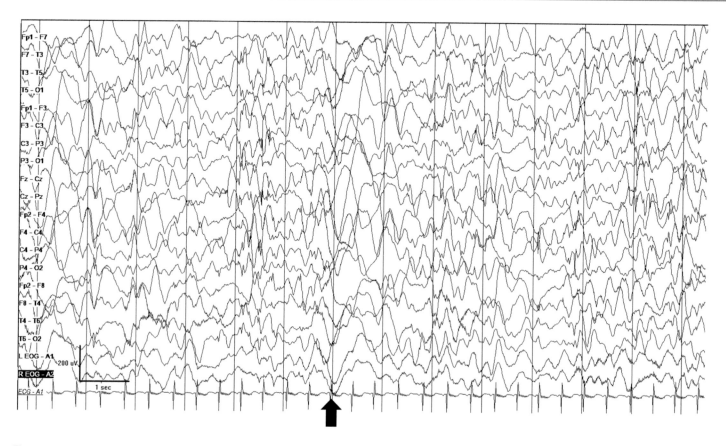

Figure 12.11 Epileptic spasm. This EEG is from a 7-month-old male with Trisomy 21, who presented with clusters of torso and head flexion. The EEG demonstrates a diffuse, high-amplitude slow wave transient with overriding fast activity (depicted by arrow) followed by 1 second relative electrodement.

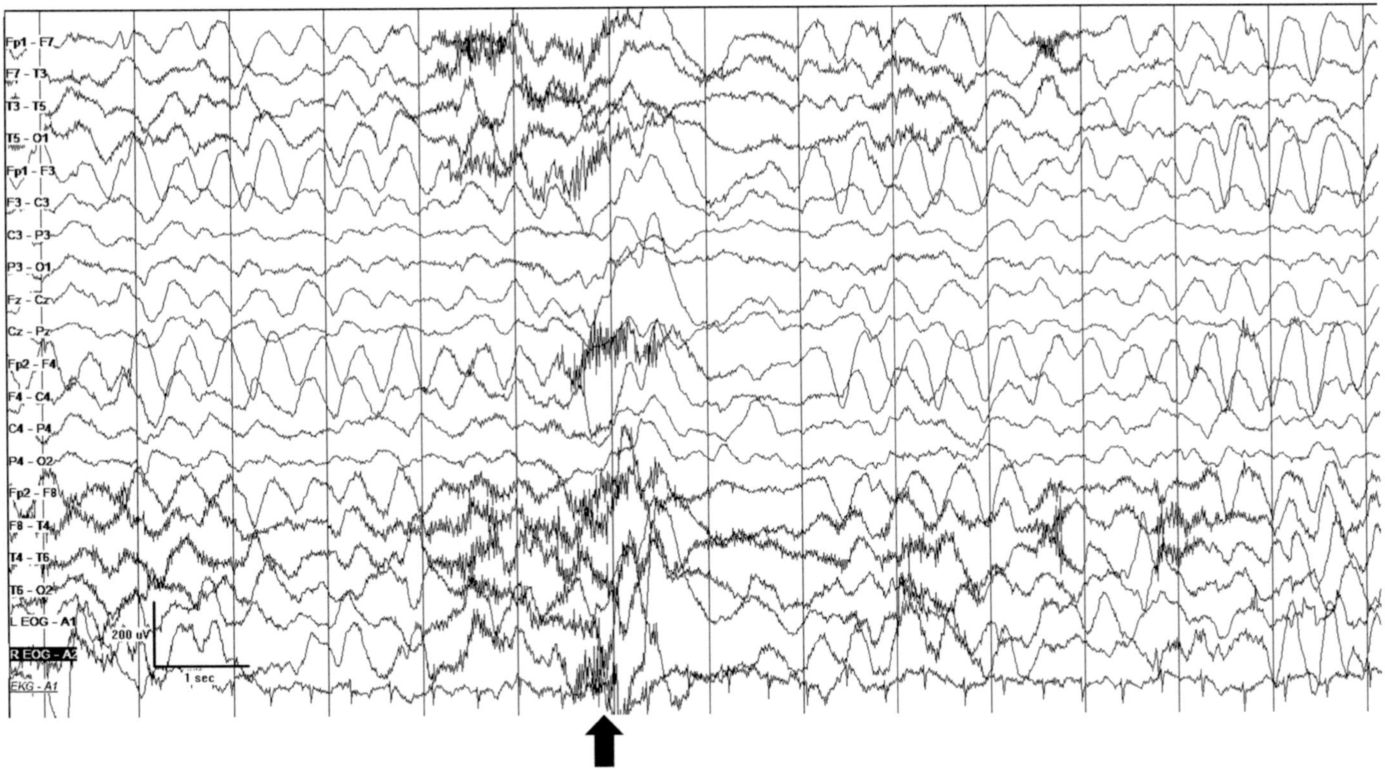

Figure 12.12   Epileptic spasm. This EEG is from a 9-month-old female with pontocerebellar hypoplasia, who presented with increasing events of bilateral arm extension or flexion. The EEG demonstrates a diffuse, very high-amplitude slow wave transient (depicted by arrow) that was correlated with an extensor spasm.

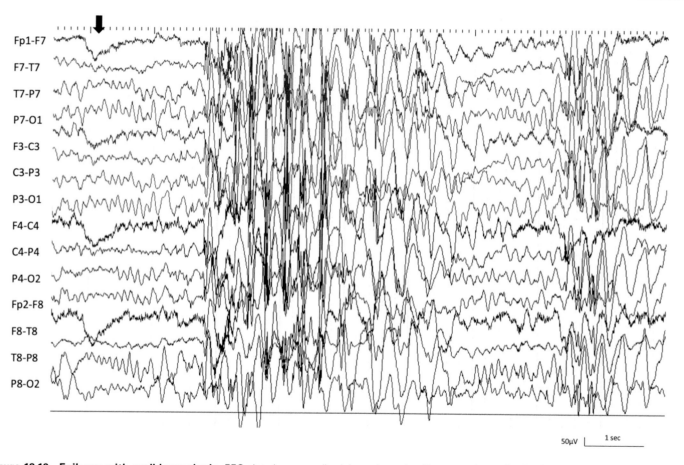

Figure 12.13   Epilepsy with eyelid myoclonia. EEG showing generalized, irregular, polyspike waves immediately after eye closure (arrow). It was associated with eyelid myoclonia without impairment of awareness.

REFERENCES

Berg AT, Berkovic SF, Brodie MJ, et al. Revised Terminology and Concepts for Organization of Seizures and Epilepsies: Report of the ILAE Commission on Classification and Terminology, 2005–2009. Epilepsia 2010;51:676–85.

Chowdhury FA, Silva R, Whatley B, Walker MC. Localization in Focal Epilepsy: A Practical Guide. Pract Neurol 2021;21:481–91.

Fisher RS, Cross JH, French JA, et al. Operational Classification of Seizure Types by the International League Against Epilepsy: Position Paper of the ILAE Commission for Classification and Terminology. Epilepsia 2017;58:522–30.

Fusco L, Vigevano F. Ictal Clinical Electroencephalographic Findings of Spasms in West Syndrome. Epilepsia 1993;34:671–78.

Hirsch LJ, Fong MWK, Leitnger M, et al. American Clinical Neurophysiology Society's Standardized Critical Care EEG Terminology: 2021 Version. J Clin Neurophysiol 2021;38:1–29.

Kellaway P, Hrachovy RA, Frost JD, et al. Precise Characterization and Quantification of Infantile Spasms. Ann Neurol 1979;6:214–18.

Mizrahi EM, Hrachovy RA. Atlas of neonatal electroencephalography. 4th Ed. New York: Demos Medical; 2016.

Nordli DR Jr, Riviello JJ Jr, Niedermeyer E. Seizures and Epilepsy in Infants to Adolescentes. In: Schomer, DL, da Silva, FHL (Eds). Niedermeyer's Electroencephalography: Basic Principles, Clinical Applications, and Related Fields, 6th Ed. Philadelphia: Lippincott Williams & Wilkins; 2011. p. 479–540.

CHAPTER 13

EEG report

Brittany Sprigg, MD

Maria Augusta Montenegro, MD, PhD

Once an electroencephalogram has been read and interpreted, a report must be generated to communicate the results to other providers. The EEG report should ideally summarize the electroencephalographic findings concisely, but with sufficient detail to allow another electroencephalographer to "visualize" the main findings and draw their own conclusions without seeing the EEG tracing. It should include sufficient information to identify the patient, some clinical background, and the conditions under which the recording was performed. It also must contain interpretation, framed to allow other providers without specific knowledge of electroencephalography to understand the study's significance. An EEG report typically consists of five main components (Tatum *et al.*, 2016):

- Technical description
- History
- EEG description
- Impression
- Clinical correlation

TECHNICAL DESCRIPTION

The technical description should delineate the type of electrode placement (the 10–20 or 10–10 system), the number of electrodes used, and whether additional electrodes were included (T1/T2, sphenoidal, subtemporal, eye movement electrodes, etc.). It also needs to mention if there was any modification of the 10–20 system and whether there is a channel with electrocardiogram (EKG).

Technical parameters such as duration of the recording, filters, and time constant used should also be described in this section. In addition, this section should contain the activation methods used, if any, such as hyperventilation, sleep deprivation, or intermittent photic stimulation.

HISTORY

The patient history should be brief and contain the patient's name, age, gender, relevant clinical information, and the reason for obtaining the EEG. Any neurotropic medications, especially sedatives or antiseizure medications, should be documented.

EEG DESCRIPTION

The description of the EEG should include both normal and abnormal findings, with subsections typically devoted to the background, interictal abnormalities, and ictal or clinical events of concern.

The background activity should be described in terms of predominant amplitudes and frequencies and should be differentiated by the state of consciousness where state changes occur during the study. A typical "awake" background description should include should include the presence or absence of features such as the anterior-posterior gradient, in which amplitudes increase and frequencies decrease from anterior to posterior leads, and the posterior dominant rhythm, including frequency, amplitude, and reactivity to eye-opening (**Figures 13.1–13.3**). A typical "asleep" background description should include which stages of sleep were observed and relevant characteristic features, such as sleep spindles and K-complexes for stage N2 and increased proportion of delta frequencies in stage N3.

Background amplitude does not necessarily need to be described in microvolts, and the wave measurement should be done from peak to trough (not peak to baseline). The American Clinical Neurophysiology Society recommends the following descriptors (Hirsch *et al.*, 2021):

- Suppressed: <10 µV
- Low: <11–20 µV
- Normal: 50–149 µV
- High: ≥150 µV

Many departments have their own established labels and parameters such as very low, low, medium, high, or very high amplitude are considered acceptable at most centers.

It is important to comment on interhemispheric symmetry and synchrony as well as any focal areas of frequency or amplitude differences. Interhemispheric symmetry applies only to the wave amplitude and frequency (**Figure 13.4**; Hirsch *et al.*, 2021):

- Mild asymmetry: Asymmetry <50% in amplitude on referential montage or frequency 0.5–1 Hz.
- Marked asymmetry: Asymmetry ≥50% in voltage or >1 Hz in frequency.

Synchrony refers to the presence of activity simultaneously in the two hemispheres (**Figure 13.5**).

The subsection on interictal findings should include any non-seizure abnormal epileptiform activity. It should be classified according to its morphology (spike, sharp wave, spike-and-slow-wave complex, sharp-and-slow-wave complex, slow wave, sharply

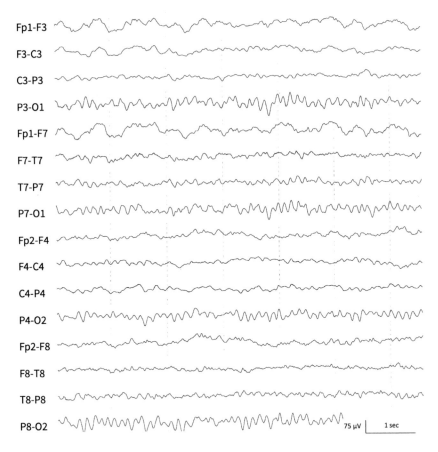

Figure 13.1 Anterior posterior gradient. EEG of a 4-year-old girl during wakefulness showing a normal anterior posterior gradient and posterior dominant rhythm of 9 Hz.

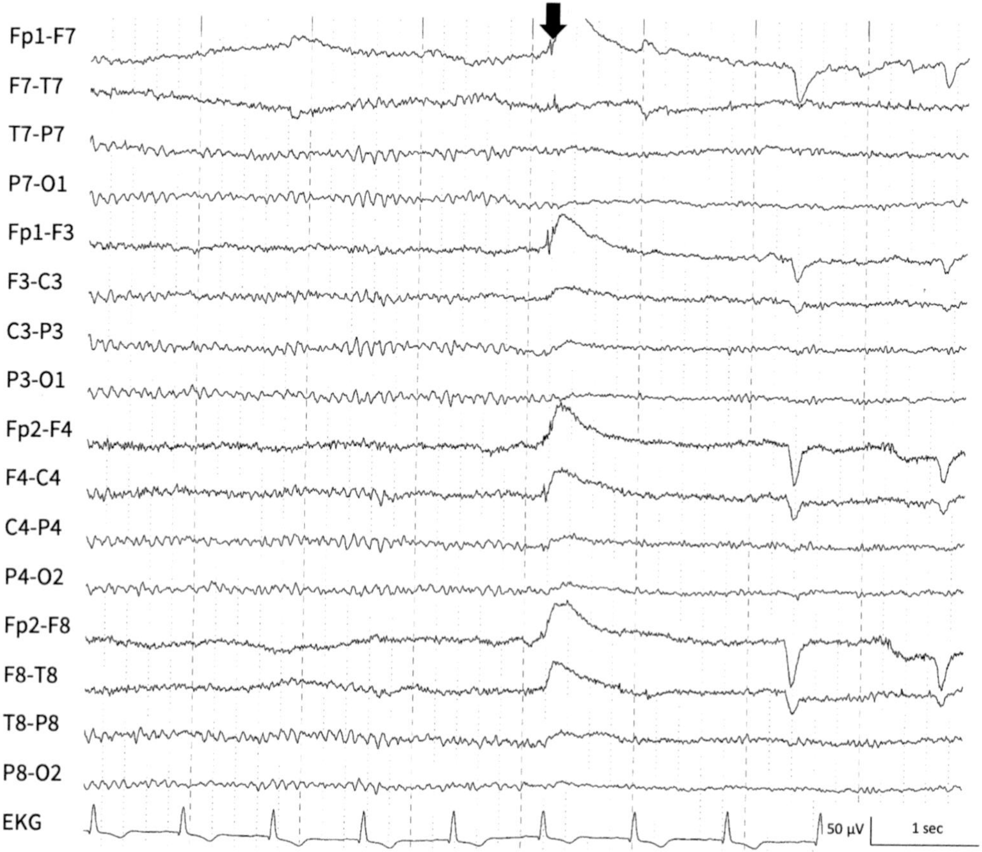

Figure 13.2   Posterior dominant rhythm reactivity. EEG showing posterior dominant rhythm attenuation after eye-opening (arrow).

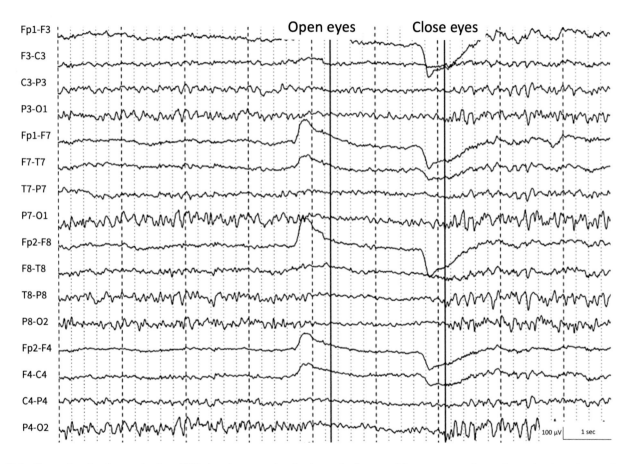

Figure 13.3   Posterior dominant rhythm. EEG showing posterior dominant rhythm reactivity to eye-opening and anterior posterior gradient.

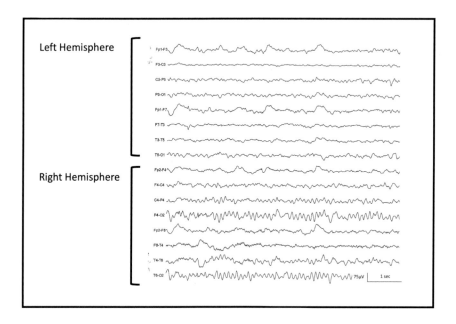

Figure 13.4 **Amplitude asymmetry**. EEG showing inter-hemispheric asymmetry, characterized by right hemisphere amplitude of more than 50% of the left hemisphere amplitude.

contoured wave; **Figure 13.6**). Its location in relation to the cerebral lobes and electrodes should be specified (where the potential has maximum negativity, phase reversal, or equipotentiality).

The frequency and the morphology (irregular or regular) of spike-wave or sharp-wave complexes should also be included in the report (**Figures 13.7–13.9**). Voltage measurement should also be done from peak to trough (not peak to baseline), and the

American Clinical Neurophysiology Society guidelines suggest the following classifications (Hirsch *et al.*, 2021):

- Very low: <20 µV
- Low: 20–49 µV
- Medium: 50–149 µV
- High: ≥150 µV

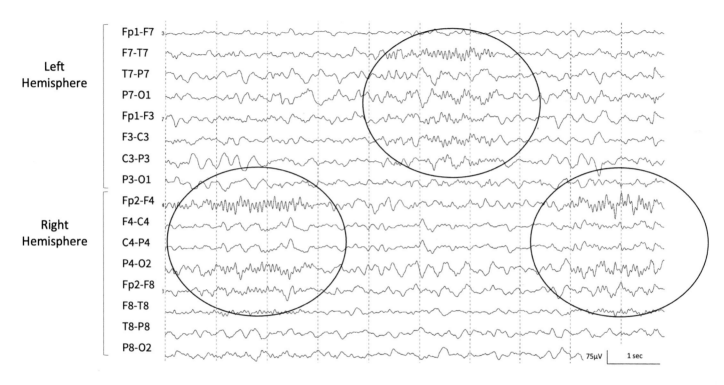

Figure 13.5   Asynchrony. EEG of a 7-month-old baby girl during sleep showing age-appropriate spindles asynchrony.

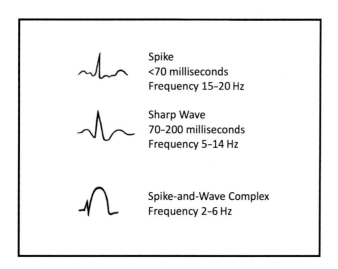

Figure 13.6 Types of epileptiform discharges. Note the morphology, frequency, and duration of each type of epileptiform activity: Spikes, sharp waves, and spike-wave complexes.

The frequency of epileptiform discharges should also be noted. Suggested parameters are (Hirsch *et al.*, 2021):

a.   Abundant (≥1 per 10 seconds).

b.   Frequent (≥1/minute, less than one in 10 seconds).

c.   Occasional (≥1 hour, but less than 1/minute).

d.   Rare (<1/hour).

As with background descriptors, many centers have their own standardized groupings for discharge voltages and prevalence, and

it is important to be aware of this terminology. Because routine EEGs frequently last less than 1 hour, we suggest the parameters below:

a.   Extremely rare (1–2 times per recording)

b.   Rare (3–5 times per recording)

c.   Recurrent (1–10 times per minute)

d.   Frequent (3–5 per 10 second page)

e.   Very frequent (6–10 per 10 second page)

f.   Abundant (>10 per page)

When an epileptiform abnormality occurs in both hemispheres, it should be noted whether it occurs independently, synchronously, or both (**Figure 13.10**). Multifocal should be used if the epileptiform activity is present in at least three independent areas with at least one in each cerebral hemisphere (Hirsch *et al.*, 2021).

A note should be included about any intensification of abnormalities by activation procedures (hyperventilation, intermittent photic stimulation or sleep; **Figures 13.11–13.13**). **Table 13.1** shows the most common descriptive terms used in the EEG report.

After the interictal findings, if a seizure is recorded, its electrographic and clinical characteristics should be described in detail, including:

● Time of electrographic onset.

● Time of clinical onset.

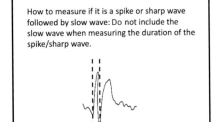

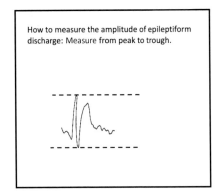

Figure 13.7   Wave measurements. The duration of the spike or sharp wave should be measured without including the following slow wave. The amplitude of the wave should be measured from peak to trough.

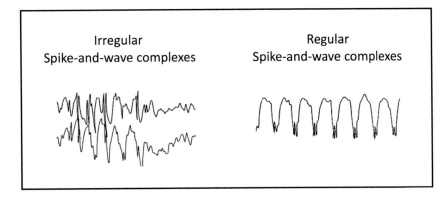

Figure 13.8   Type of spike-wave complex. It is usually associated with generalized epilepsies, the slow wave has a higher amplitude than the spike, and they are classified according to their morphology: Irregular (different morphology) and regular (same morphology in each channel).

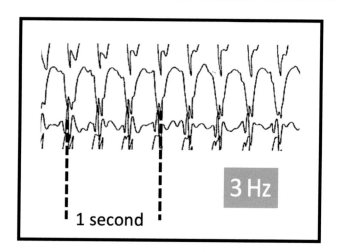

Figure 13.9 Spike and wave complex. The figure shows how to measure the frequency of spike-wave complexes.

- Wave morphology and amplitude at onset, evolution into faster frequencies and higher amplitude.
- Localization.
- Duration.
- Clinical characteristics.

Electrographic seizures are defined as rhythmic discharges lasting at least 10 seconds with at least one of the characteristics: a) Sustained spike-wave discharges with a frequency ≥2.5 Hz; or b) Evolving ictal activity with a dynamic evolution in time and space (Hirsch *et al.*, 2021).

Table 13.1   Most common descriptive terms used in the EEG report

Type of wave	Characteristics
Periodic	Uniform wave repetition (at least six cycles), with regular interval between them.
Rhythmic delta activity	Uniform delta wave repetition (<4 Hz), without interval between them.
Discharge	Waves lasting <0.5 seconds, regardless of the number of phases, or waves ≥5 seconds with no more than three phases.
Burst	Waves should last ≥5 seconds and have at least four phases.
Burst-attenuation	Bursts of generalized activity, followed by background attenuation of at least 50% of its amplitude (should be higher than ≥10 μV, which would be a suppression).
Burst-suppression	Bursts of generalized activity, followed by background suppression ≤10 μV.
Brief rhythmic discharge (Yoo *et al.*, 2017)	Focal or generalized rhythmic activity, at least six waves, lasting ≥0.5 to <10 seconds. Must have at least one of the following: • Evolution. • Similar morphology and location to patient's interictal discharges or seizures. • Sharply contoured and rhythmic.

Source: Hirsch *et al.*, (2021).

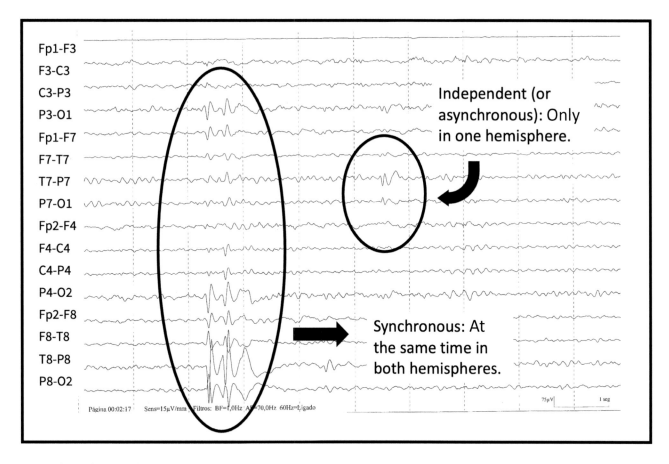

Figure 13.10 Classification of epileptiform discharges. EEG showing epileptiform discharges in a patient with self-limited epilepsy with centrotemporal spikes. Note that there are both synchronous and asynchronous discharges.

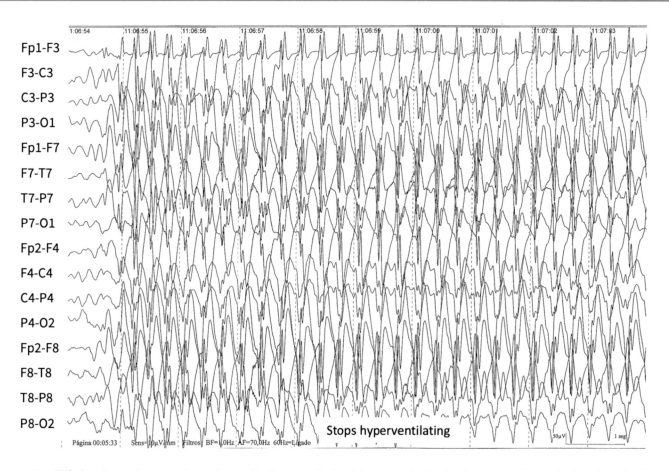

Figure 13.11   EEG showing an absence seizure triggered by hyperventilation. It is characterized by the abrupt onset of generalized regular 3 Hz spike-wave complexes, with a total duration of 17 seconds. *(Continued)*

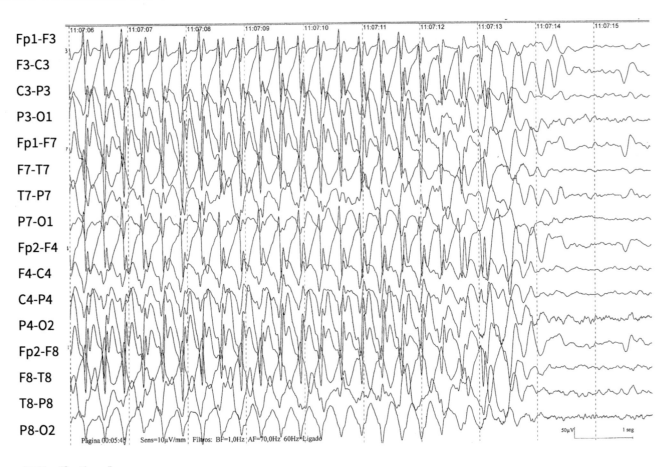

Figure 13.11 *(Continued)*

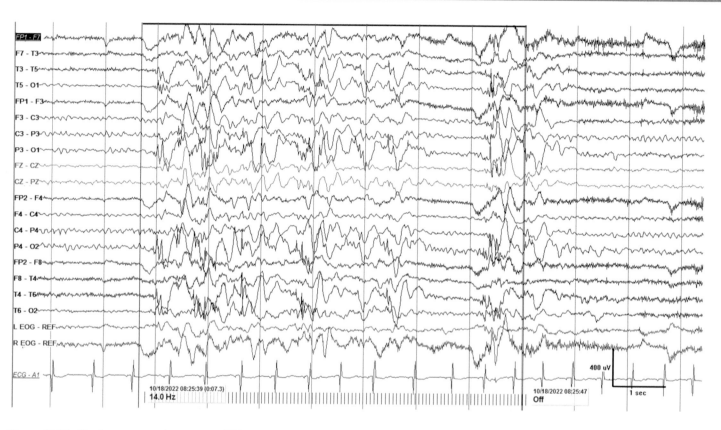

Figure 13.12 Photoparoxysmal response. EEG showing generalized irregular polyspike-wave discharges during 14 Hz intermittent photic stimulation in a patient idiopathic generalized epilepsy.

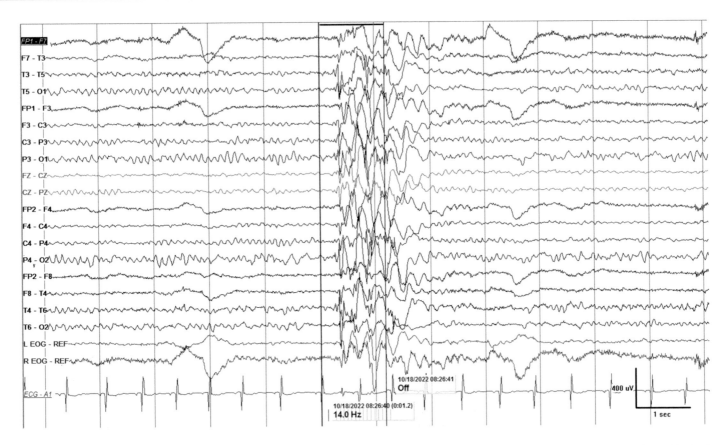

Figure 13.13   Photoparoxysmal response. EEG from the same patient showing generalized irregular spike-wave complexes when the 14 Hz photic stimulation was repeated. The photic stimulation was turned off after 1 second to prevent triggering a seizure.

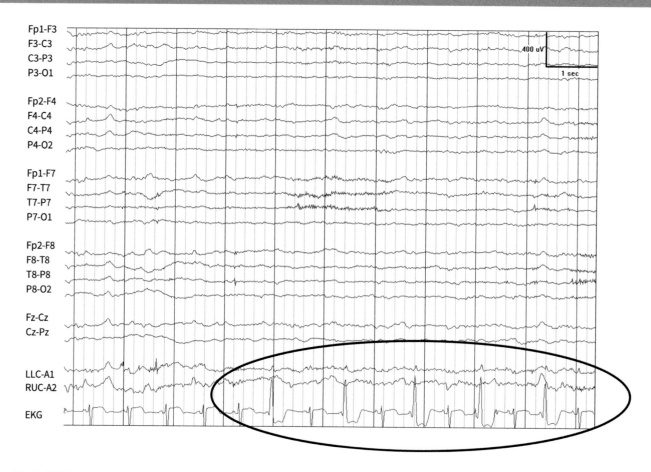

Figure 13.14   EKG abnormality. EEG showing normal findings, but the EKG channel shows abnormal QRS complexes in a boy with syncopal episodes due to Wolff-Parkinson-White syndrome.

The 10 seconds necessary to characterize an electrographic seizure is arbitrary, and some authors argue that several clinical seizures are shorter than 10 seconds at any age. Most neurophysiologists agree, however, that if a subclinical rhythmic discharge lasts 10 seconds or longer, it should be classified as an electrographic seizure. Rhythmic discharges with a shorter duration are classified as brief rhythmic discharges (BRDs; also called brief interictal/ictal rhythmic discharges: BIRDs; Pressler *et al.*, 2021).

BRDs are part of the ictal-interictal continuum, which includes discharges that are not clear if ictal or interictal. In addition to BRDs, the most common ictal-interictal continuum patterns seen in children are periodic discharges, burst suppression, rhythmic delta activity (without clear evolution), and extreme delta brush. These discharges indicate an increased potential for seizures and further neuronal injury (Riviello & Appavu, 2021).

Electrographic status epilepticus is defined as electrographic seizures lasting more than 10 minutes or more $\geq 20\%$ of 60 minutes of EEG recording (Hirsch *et al.*, 2021).

If there were non-epileptic clinical events noted during the study, they should be described, and the absence of correlating electrographic activity should be clearly noted.

Finally, a small comment about the EKG recording should also be included. This can be limited to the notation of whether EKG activity was regular in rate and rhythm. If morphological abnormalities were seen, this should be documented but need not be described in detail (**Figure 13.14**)

INTERPRETATION

The electroencephalographer's impression of the tracing is included as a reference to the physician who requested the test. It should objectively summarize the findings in such a way that another provider can understand the report, even without specific training in electroencephalography. It should start with a statement as to whether the EEG is normal or abnormal (Tatum *et al.*, 2016). It should also include the patient's state(s) of consciousness (awake, drowsy, asleep, comatose, etc.) and should go on to highlight any abnormal findings. Typically, abnormalities noted in the interpretation are listed in order of decreasing immediate clinical relevance. Technical terms of electroencephalography should be avoided in this section when possible.

CLINICAL CORRELATION

The report concludes with a mention of the findings' significance within a specific clinical picture. The explanation may vary according to the professional to whom the report is intended, especially in the case of non-neurologists. Specific therapeutic suggestions should not be included in the EEG report, but suggestions for further testing (EEG with sleep deprivation, video-EEG, cardiologic evaluation if EKG is abnormal, etc.) should be included in this section (Tatum *et al.*, 2016).

The clinical correlation should make it clear that, in some situations, an abnormal EEG does not necessarily mean cerebral abnormality or epilepsy, just as a normal EEG does not rule out the presence of brain pathology.

REFERENCES

Hirsch LJ, Fong MWK, Leitnger M, et al. American Clinical Neurophysiology Society's Standardized Critical Care EEG Terminology: 2021 Version. J Clin Neurophysiol 2021;38:1–29.

Pressler RM, Cilio MR, Mizrahi EM, et al. The ILAE Classification of Seizures and the Epilepsies: Modification for Seizures in the Neonate. Position Paper by the ILAE Task Force on Neonatal Seizures. Epilepsia 2021;62:615–28.

Riviello JJ Jr, Appavu B. Multimodal monitoring and the ictal-interictal continuum. In: Atlas of Pediatric and Neonatal ICU EEG. Sansevere AJ, Harrar DB (eds). Springer Publishing Company, Danver 2021.

Tatum WO, Olga S, Ochoa JG, et al. American Clinical Neurophysiology Society Guideline 7: Guidelines for EEG Reporting. J Clin Neurophysiol 2016;33:328–32.

Yoo JY, Marcuse LV, Fields MC, et al. Brief potentially ictal rhythmic discharges [B(I)RDs] in noncritically ill adults. J Clin Neurophysiol 2017;34:222–29.

Index

Note: Locators in *italics* represent figures and **bold** indicate tables in the text.